SHARP SCRATCH

Deborah Jay

Dedication

For everyone fighting invisible battles

&

To everyone helping me fight mine

Preface

On 13th January 2015, I went into hospital for a hysterectomy – technical term *hysterectomy with bilateral salpingo-oophorectomy,* which means the fallopian tubes (salpingectomy), womb, cervix and ovaries (oophorectomy) are removed. This operation was to eliminate doubt about a 'suspect mass', a legacy after thirty years of severe endometriosis and bowel disease, during which time I'd undergone in excess of thirty operations and procedures. The hysterectomy proved to be extremely complex, with serious complications and has left me with life-changing consequences. It's been a seven-year journey to date and I wanted to share it with anyone who's been plunged into a type of hell you didn't even know existed . . .

The Back Story

I was born in 1960 and had a happy and fairly healthy childhood, though I do recall having scarlet fever when I was 10 and had to stay off school for several months. School work was sent home to me and books were returned and burned to avoid contamination, making me feel like I had the plague! I then had my tonsils out at 12 and that was about it. All very boring and fairly normal. I was an only child until I was 12 years 7 months old, when my mother had another baby, a little girl and a sister for me, at last.

When I was nineteen, I met Andrew. He was six years older than me and from my hometown but he had joined the Navy when he was just 16, so had been living away and travelling the world. We married when I was just 20 and on my 21st birthday, we moved to married quarters in Plymouth. Six months later, the Falklands War started and he went away indefinitely.

I moved home as I couldn't settle, my Nan was terminally ill, and I missed my family so much. I soon gained employment in a bank and in 1984 we had a lovely little daughter. Unbeknown to me until the day I went into labour, the baby was breech. But in those days, you had to just get on with it, no husband as he was at sea, only my very stressed mother who was not a woman of words. I was, however, reassured that as I had large feet, I'd be fine - the rationale being I also had a large pelvis! It was a very long and difficult labour, requiring me to be cut rather hastily, but our beautiful daughter eventually came into the world a healthy 8lbs and I instantly fell in love with her.

We had a happy life and looked forward to Andrew's weekend leaves when we would spend family time together.

When Annie was about 1 year old, I noticed I was becoming very constipated. I could go several weeks without a bowel motion, despite eating all the right things and eventually resorting to laxatives. Doctors' visits were numerous, yet pointless, as I was told repeatedly to eat oranges, drink more water, or try and relax. I think I was even called a 'neurotic mum' by one GP which was neither helpful nor true. They soon took notice, however, when I started losing copious amounts of blood. Tests eventually revealed I was suffering from proctitis which is inflammation in the rectum.

As consultant visits became more frequent, he prescribed steroid drugs in an attempt to dampen down the inflammation. Initially, these proved to be effective but were a 'double edged sword', resulting in numerous side effects. The most distressing for me was the dreaded 'moon face' whereby fat and fluid collects around your cheeks. I found this quite embarrassing to deal with and, as time went on, their efficacy diminished. My consultant explained the next step would be to try another drug or surgery - a colostomy was mentioned which bothered me greatly.

I decided to soldier on and tried the drug, which was called Sulfasalazine, in the hope it would bring about a remission. Whilst it helped to a certain degree, it did not stop the disease from progressing.

Life became difficult as I struggled to cope with this awful disease which was slowly creeping its way up my colon. On the daily bus journey to work, I would be praying I wouldn't have an accident as the diarrhoea had become unrelenting. I hadn't been in my job that long and they were not very understanding. After all, in those days, bowel issues were not discussed openly. I'd arrive at the office and have to run up three flights of stairs to the only toilet, before starting a day's work, putting on a brave face and hoping my bowels would behave.

Like anyone with a chronic debilitating illness, I struggled. Andrew was away, I had a busy toddler to look after and only my parents to lean on. My mother, in particular, also struggled with the prospect of me having an illness and she used to refer to it as 'my condition'. Looking back, I never realised how much my mother had to deal with but she never wavered or let me down.

I had to spend so much time in the bathroom with Annie in tow. I remember my bathroom had a blue carpet and as she grew up, Annie refused to use anyone's loo unless it had a blue carpet! I tried to hide a lot of the problems from her and luckily, she was very happy to stay with her Nanni and Grampy, as my hospital stays became more and more frequent.

I was also having to take sick leave from work which added to my distress. I had a strong work ethic, but I knew I wasn't coping. I had told my supervisor that a stoma bag had been mentioned to relieve my symptoms and he didn't really pass comment. I remember one day coming back from lunch early, only to witness him prancing about the office with a carrier bag tied to his front, telling all the other staff that I was going to have a bag because I had a poop problem. I realised then my days there were numbered. I left shortly afterwards - I was upset, of course, but also relieved to have one less thing to worry about.

As my illness progressed, the fear of surgery hung heavily over me. I was 27, with a little girl and an absent husband. I was devastated.

Soon, I was admitted to hospital with an uncontrollable flare up. I had an abscess in my armpit, was having relentless bloody diarrhoea every day and no sooner had they transfused me than I'd be anaemic again.

I started losing dramatic amounts of weight and they decided to try steroids in an attempt to bring things under control. But the steroids were not working quickly enough, in reality nothing was working. I'd been in hospital for several weeks and was desperate to get home to Annie who was now aged three. I knew my parents were doing a great job looking after her, but it broke my heart having to say goodbye after her visits. She was often tearful and calling for me as my parents left the ward to take her home, I was assured her distress was very short lived but that was little consolation to me.

After being extremely unwell for a few weeks, it was discovered I was, in fact, fourteen weeks pregnant, which was what had caused the disease to go into a massive flareup! Andrew was granted compassionate leave as he was told my life was at risk unless I terminated the pregnancy. I had a three-year-old at home who needed me, and I was faced with an impossible decision - abort the pregnancy or risk possible death.

I was in a very bad place, and I took to wandering the wards, looking for someone to tell me what to do. In those days, there was no support or counselling – you were just left to it. The doctors felt I should terminate as apart from the effects on my health, I'd had multiple X-rays and so many drugs that it was likely the foetus could have been damaged. They also said that if I decided to proceed with the pregnancy and survived, I would have to have a colostomy, whereas, if I terminated, it was quite likely things would settle down, thereby sparing me radical surgery.

I decided to terminate the pregnancy as I was desperate to get better for my little girl and hated the thought of leaving her motherless. Arrangements were put in place and the termination was planned for the following week. I was heartbroken. I never conceived again, I felt it was my punishment. To make matters worse, the flare up didn't settle down and a few months later, I had a colostomy. I was 27 years old and felt mutilated. I remember my dad putting his arms around me after my colostomy saying, 'What have they done to you?' We both cried.

More bad news followed as the histology revealed it looked more like Crohn's colitis than ulcerative colitis, but there was some uncertainty. Crohn's disease can affect any part of your alimentary canal from your mouth to your anus, whereas in those days, ulcerative colitis was thought to be less serious as it only affected your colon and therefore could be 'cured', albeit by the removal of the colon and the formation of an ileostomy.

So, I now felt devastated that, despite losing the baby and having a colostomy, I was never likely to get better as the disease could recur at any time. In those days, there was no internet. I used to lurk in WH Smith's and read medical books about Crohn's, desperate to find some positivity but there was none. This disease was terrifying - I really felt my life was over.

I worried constantly about Annie, terrified something would happen to me and she would have to grow up without me. I remember, when she was three, I used to buy clothes aged eight and store them in her wardrobe in case her future didn't include me. I knew she would be absolutely loved and cherished by her dad and the family but the thought of not being there for her was, understandably, pure torture. I used to pray to God to let me live until she was eighteen, thinking naïvely it would somehow be easier to have to say goodbye to her, but once a mother, always a mother and it never gets easier. My anxiety was constantly fuelled by my poor health, to the point I became afraid of the future rather than embracing it, which was not helping matters. Andrew was (and remains) a fixer and we were unable to forge a connection on this. The best he could offer was 'At least it's not cancer' which somehow invalidated my feelings and experiences.

My health, however, did improve somewhat but it wasn't long before symptoms returned and in 1989, they decided to perform an ileostomy. The diagnosis changed again to ulcerative colitis, and I was really glad to be free of that toxic colon that had plagued me for so many years. They had left the rectal stump *in situ* and said 'it would burn itself out' which, looking back, seems odd advice as I don't think any inflammatory bowel disease does this. I didn't question it (in those days, you never questioned doctors) and tried to get on with my life.

Within a few months, I was so much better and my health was improving daily as I got stronger and stronger. By now, Andrew had left the Royal Navy and had joined the police force and I had started working for the local authority. Life was good! I adapted really well to having a stoma and it gave me back my health. I completely embraced it and it never stopped me doing anything.

Just a year or so later, I became unwell again with abdominal pain that seemed to be linked to my menstrual cycle. Again, more doctors and more tests and I was told it was adhesions, a recurrence of the bowel disease or good old stress. I eventually had an MRI of my pelvis, and the results were pretty terrifying. I was told I had a suspect mass and it looked like ovarian cancer. Exploratory surgery quickly followed, and I was diagnosed, not with cancer, but with severe endometriosis. Endometriosis is the name given to the condition where cells, like the ones in the lining of the womb (uterus), are found elsewhere in the body. It is a chronic and debilitating condition that causes pain, fatigue and many other problems. My consultant said it was the worst he had ever seen. They were unable to do anything much, apart from confirm the origins of the mass (benign fibroma) and close me back up. I was told I'd be treated conservatively for the endometriosis as it was so extensive and obliterated my whole pelvis, essentially gluing everything together.

A week after this operation, I had a complete bowel obstruction which was the worst experience of my life to date. The pain was immeasurable and coupled with faecal vomiting, the whole event really was horrific. I had to go back to theatre where they tried to untangle the glued-up mess that was my small bowel. I woke up wrapped in a foil blanket and discovered Andrew and my parents had been told it was touch and go. The surgeons had been unable to clear the blockage completely but thought it may resolve itself in time. I stayed in hospital for a month being vein-fed and thankfully my gut started working again. I returned to work shortly after, determined this was not going to affect me for one minute longer than necessary.

When I went for my follow up consultation with the gynaecologist a few weeks later, he told me the stark reality of the severity of the endometriosis. He explained it was so extensive that, coupled with the bowel obstruction I'd experienced after the last operation, he would never operate on me again unless my life was at risk. He said the condition would be managed conservatively with drugs to essentially bring on the menopause. These drugs could have unwanted androgenic side effects like facial hair, a deepening voice and acne. I was mortified but realised I had no choice. As it happened, I didn't develop any of these side effects but what I did have were fluid collections deep in the pelvic cavity.

So, in 1991, I started a twenty-year journey of living with this manifestation of severe endometriosis which was really hard going and affected every aspect of my life.

Living with a chronic illness is a learning process and I found it as difficult then to accept my limitations, as I do now. Work and homelife had to be carefully managed to avoid me becoming burnt out, but by his own admission, Andrew had little empathy for this having never experienced ill health himself. A main bone of contention was holidays. We never had the luxury of booking anything in advance and just had to go when we could. This became normal life for us but it really got him down as he craved excitement and spontaneity, whereas I just wanted to be well, preferring to stay where I felt safe, at home.

Apart from the pain, exhaustion, bleeding, and the general feeling of malaise that chronic illness dishes out, the cysts required surgical intervention at least once a year, when they reached a size, usually around 11cm, that caused me pain. This always involved a general anaesthetic and a trip to theatre where the surgeon would insert a catheter-type instrument up through the top of my vagina, or through my abdominal wall, and burst the cyst. The drains were then left in and I'd wake up with two catheters coming out of me, connected to drainage bags which were invariably full of black gunk. All of this became worryingly routine. I always bounced back and used to return to work and normality in no time. Yes, I was always in pain but that was normal, wasn't it? Little did I realise the monster these repeated procedures were creating within me.

Chapter 1

2010

The year of my Big Birthday. I was to be fifty in October. My twenties, thirties and forties had been plagued by illness, but things were finally better. The aspirations of the cysts were less frequent now that the menopause had arrived. The gynaecologist explained that endometriosis is driven by oestrogen and so the cessation of my periods was to be my panacea.

We deliberated what to do for this special milestone birthday, and eventually decided on a house party. I liked organising such things but even then, I found it quite stressful, trying to decide who to invite etc, factoring in the available space in our small bungalow. Never one to make things easy for myself, I finally decided on a two-tier party. I asked my work friends and their children to an afternoon tea at 4pm and then a drinks and nibbles party for my family at 8pm. The rationale being the work friends would go before the family arrived. Of course, it didn't work out like that and it ended up being quite chaotic but lots of fun. I realised it was time to draw things to a close when my aunty took a tumble and bashed her head on the patio door and our neighbour (who was a vicar) had partaken of way too much red wine and had to be escorted home by my equally drunk mother!

At midnight, after a bit of tidying, we collapsed in a heap on the sofa vowing 'never again' but knowing it had actually gone very well and we went to bed in a state of happy exhaustion.

I was still having regular scans and by now, I'd been classed as 'complex', with only a few radiographers prepared to scan me for fear of missing something. On more than one occasion, it had been suggested by one of these radiographers that I should maybe get a second opinion on these cysts, as repeatedly aspirating the same area and puncturing the same tissue over and over again wasn't really the best idea and could be causing untold damage. I explained that the gynaecologist felt this was the best course of action, considering my frozen pelvis. A 'frozen pelvis' usually refers to the situation where there has been marked inflammation within the pelvic tissues, the most common culprit being endometriosis. The fact he had aspirated these cysts in excess of twenty times must be acceptable and safe, mustn't it, as he was the consultant, the expert? There was some confusion as to what the cysts were. They had been given several names – pseudo cysts, peritoneal cysts, ovarian cysts – it didn't matter to me, I completely trusted my consultant. He said it was the safest way of dealing with them and I was doing ok with his method. He would not even consider a hysterectomy as he said it would be so easy to make things much worse. I accepted this as the drainage of the cysts relieved me of pain and I was able to get back to work and get on with life, albeit a scaled down version of the life we had hoped for.

I continued to work full time. My employer – local government - was very supportive and made several adjustments to my working day to help me manage my condition. Fatigue was a problem but I loved my job and gave it my all. My life revolved around my family and my job. Two little boys had also come into our world in 2009 when my sister had twins. I loved them like my own and they became, and remain, a big part of our life.

Life rumbled on. I was still having regular surveillance on my pelvis and rectal stump, I was still classed as complex and as a complication for me, my long-term gynaecologist was retiring, after looking after me for over twenty years. He referred me to a colleague who had vast experience in more complex cases like mine. I attended an ultrasound scan appointment with the new doctor and he expressed concern at the suspect mass. Even though my old consultant had explained everything to him about my history and risks of surgery, he still felt a hysterectomy was the only way to be sure what we were dealing with. I was stunned. I'd spent years being told to avoid any kind of invasive surgery owing to the risks and now it seemed it was my only option to have peace of mind as to exactly what was going on in my pelvis!

Plus of course, I still had my rectal stump. Usually, a detached rectal stump is removed after about ten years as they then become a cancer risk. Mine had been there for over thirty years. So, the plan was a double whammy. They would remove my rectum at the same time as performing the hysterectomy. I was introduced to the colorectal surgeon and we scheduled the operation for the 'near future', to give me time to lose some weight and get fit. I reluctantly agreed and was glad I had some time to come to terms with it all. The alternative to surgery would be constant surveillance on both the suspect mass, plus the rectal stump. As my pelvis was so complex, imaging was becoming unreliable and my consultant felt if something sinister did develop, it could be missed. I couldn't take that chance. Andrew and I discussed this with the family so everyone knew my situation and I explained the position to my employers. I now had to get fit and get some positivity in my head.

Then, without warning, my mother had a massive brain haemorrhage.

CHAPTER 2

2012

My sister, who is thirteen years younger than me, was reaching forty and had planned a foreign holiday to get away from all the attention. I have no idea why, she looks great - much younger than her years and, much to my annoyance, is frequently mistaken for my daughter! The night before her birthday, we went to her house where we all shared a few bottles of wine to celebrate her big birthday and my mother was there with us and appeared in fine fettle. The twins gave their mother a cake and all was well in our world.

The next day my sister, the twins and Annie left for the airport to catch their flight to Spain. My sister sent me a text to say my mother hadn't turned up as expected to see them off which was not like her, so later that day, I drove the short journey to her house. My mother was seventy-three and fiercely independent. She had worked until very recently and looked after herself without needing any help. In fact, she helped my sister a lot with the twins. She had high blood pressure and we had many conversations about her smoking and her inability to take the blood pressure medication which made her feel very unwell. She was monitored by her GP who had changed her medication a few months previously. I arrived at her house and the curtains were shut, it was 2pm, my stomach churned. My mother was a creature of habit, up and dressed early, then out and about or helping my sister, that was her routine. Her car was outside and the door was locked. I had a key so opened the door and could see the back kitchen curtains were also closed This did not bode well. I walked the few steps to the parlour and could see her slumped in the chair. I thought she was dead. I ran to her and quickly realised she was still alive, but something was seriously amiss. I was thinking a stroke possibly. The ambulance was called and I phoned a family member to help. The paramedics did their checks and rushed her to hospital. I followed in my car. Andrew eventually arrived, he'd been working and out of mobile contact.

Several hours later, we were told she had had a posterior fossa brain haemorrhage and was unlikely to survive the night. My sister, daughter and the twins had arrived in Spain and I had yet to tell them the news. We sat with my mother and a few hours later, we had a visit from the consultant to say she was being transferred to the neurological unit in City Hospital. Having seen her CT scan, they now felt this would be the best place to deal with this kind of brain injury. My mother went by ambulance and we made the eighty-mile journey by car. Before doing so, we called at her house to make sure it was secure and to pick up a few things for her. I looked in the fridge and saw seven loaves of bread, the cupboard was full of jars of coffee and tinned peas, but nothing else. Headache tablets seemed to be everywhere, with no sign of any blood pressure medication. What had been going on here? It was looking increasingly like she had been having problems with her memory and had been taking lots of pain killers. As for her blood pressure tablets, there were none to be found.

It was 4am when we arrived at the hospital. It was vast and nothing like we were used to. We eventually found the neurological unit where my mother had been admitted, now semi-conscious and stable. They told us that she would be closely observed overnight but they didn't feel she was in any immediate danger so told us to go home and come back in the morning. We drove the eighty miles home in silence, both exhausted. I didn't tell my sister and daughter the full story, just the bare outline, and told them to enjoy their holiday, which of course, they didn't.

My mother stayed in hospital for nine months. It was a torrid time for us making the daily three-hour round trip to find my mother unresponsive or abusive. There was no real progress or pattern to her behaviour. Sometimes she knew us, sometimes she didn't, sometimes she cried, other times she threw things and shouted foul language. My mother had never been abusive to us and we didn't recognise this person who had taken over her mind. She hallucinated about dead children in her bed or she thought she was on a sinking cruise ship. On her calmer days, she used to ask me to comb her hair and tell her nice stories about the twins, which caused tears to stream down her face. It was all so sad I could barely handle it but I had no choice.

After several months in hospital on very powerful anti-psychotic drugs, she deteriorated quite fast and the doctors discovered she'd had a bilateral subdural haematoma which occurs when a blood vessel in the space between the skull and the brain (the subdural space) is damaged, thereby creating massive pressure.

I'm not really sure exactly when the injury happened. She had had several falls while in the hospital but the haematoma was only picked up when she suddenly deteriorated and a further CT of her head was carried out. Following this, she became increasingly aggressive, and I had a phone call telling me she had given a nurse a black eye. It was at this point that the decision was made to operate and insert shunts to relieve the pressure.

Sadly, this made things worse, and she alternated between periods of aggression and extreme drowsiness but she never came back to us, at least not properly. The damage had been quite extensive and permanent, meaning she would most likely need 24-hour care.

Several assessments later, it was obvious to the hospital that she would have to go into a nursing home. We weren't happy with this and had to fight every step of the way to avoid it, eventually managing to get her into a rehab unit where she stayed for a further three months, undergoing continual assessment. She improved somewhat and they agreed to work towards the ultimate goal of her returning to her own home, with the help of carers and family, of course.

The stress and trauma took its toll on all of us, and my health deteriorated. I had become seriously depressed and anxious about my mother, my health, and life in general. We decided to try and go away before my mother was discharged from the rehab unit. I say 'we'; it was always Andrew who had itchy feet about travel. But arranging it all was a welcome distraction once we had decided on Malta. My friends and family encouraged me to take this leap of faith and have some much-needed rest, recuperation and FUN.

We arrived in Malta on a beautiful day in late September. As we stepped off the plane, the heat hit me, even though on Malta's scale, this was nothing. We made the short journey to our hotel on the seafront which definitely had the WOW factor. But my conscience wasn't taking a holiday! As soon as I entered the room, the familiar feeling of guilt hit me, guilt at leaving my mother in the rehab unit and guilt at leaving my sister and daughter to cope with any queries. Why did I feel responsible for everyone else's happiness? It was a burden I'd carried all my life. However, I knew I wouldn't have seen her anyway, even if I'd been at home. As she'd only just been admitted to the rehab unit, we had been told not to visit for a few weeks to enable her to settle in. So, I tried to put this to one side for the next week. Andrew needed some of me too and I needed to remember that life existed outside the stress and trauma of the past few months. We sat on the balcony taking in the view – the sun sparkled on the azure waters of the Mediterranean and we sipped on ice-cold cocktails. Life suddenly felt very different from just a few days before and I felt calm and relaxed. But the guilt was never far away - I felt I didn't deserve any happiness whilst my mother was having such an awful time.

We spent the week walking, talking and relaxing. We went on a day trip to Valletta, which was like stepping back in time as we took in the amazing sights of this architectural jewel. Andrew had spent a few years based in Malta when he was in the Navy and as we stopped for a much-needed drink in the sunshine, he reminisced about days gone by. The heat of the day trapped within the city walls meant we were both glad to get on the ferry for the short cooling journey back to Sliema. It was so good not to be talking about health issues like subdural haematoma, brain injuries and my own problems, of course, but still thoughts of my mother seeped into my mind with crushing regularity.

The week passed away too quickly and soon our holiday was over. The night before we left, we had a wonderful meal at a harbour-side restaurant. There was some kind of festival on and fireworks adorned the night sky. We both felt refreshed and rejuvenated, ready to face the world again, whatever it may bring.

We arrived home and stepped back into reality very quickly. I phoned the rehab centre for an update and they said she was 'fine'. How I disliked that word! Quite often, it meant things were anything but. However, I had to trust what they said.

There was also a letter from my consultant in relation to my recent scan. My heart thudded in my chest as I opened it, hiding it from Andrew as I didn't want to burst his post-holiday happiness bubble. It was good news – it confirmed that no changes had been identified and they were happy to keep monitoring me until my mother's situation was clearer which was a huge relief. I had felt so well in Malta that it again made me question how much the stresses and strains of life were adding to my problems. Then again, these were things that couldn't be avoided, so maybe I just needed to learn to manage things better.

At the end of 2012, I was medically retired from my job which was another massive loss. I was hoping to have returned part time but with my declining health and my impending surgery, they felt I was unable to fulfil my duties. They were undoubtedly right but it was still hard. I had worked there for twenty-three years and valued my job greatly.

My mother came out of the rehabilitation unit in the spring of 2013 and I was tasked with overseeing her care. We had managed to make some adjustments to her house to make it possible for her to come home, but we knew it wasn't going to be easy. My sister and daughter both worked full time and of course, we had the twins to look after who were by now aged four. Carers would come in three times a day, with numerous 'pop-ins' from me, my sister and daughter. We set up a rota and installed a camera to keep an eye on her, but it was very hard going. The carers were often unreliable, my mother uncooperative - she didn't accept there was anything wrong with her and resented the presence of the carers. She also wanted to go out every day which was just impossible. Her brain haemorrhage had left her right side seriously weakened and she often relied on a wheelchair. If I did manage to get her to town, she would insist on buying things she couldn't afford and shopping for food she didn't like.

One such shopping trip sticks in my mind with crushing embarrassment. Every week we went to Marks and Spencer to do some food shopping. Andrew would reluctantly accompany us as I couldn't manage the wheelchair, as at this point, my mother was still about 11 stone!

We arrived in store and she insisted on having the basket on her lap and choosing her own shopping, with Andrew following with a trolley doing her actual shopping which consisted of meals for the week. The first thing she always chose was a large French stick, which soon became a weapon of mass destruction, as it hung menacingly out of the basket. Every week I'd say, 'You don't need that, Mam,' and every week she ignored me. Sometimes I'd manage to sneak it out of the basket and replace it with a baguette but not on this particular occasion. As we went past the wine aisle, I stopped to chat to a friend. Next minute, I heard a huge crash as she used the French stick to flick several bottles of red wine onto the floor! Staff came running, thinking there had been an accident as my mother looked on laughing. All I could do was apologise but inside I was dying of embarrassment and frustration. Andrew stormed off muttering 'Never again!' to anyone who'd listen and as usual, I was left to deal with it all.

My mother had forgotten the incident within minutes, whereas I realised that maybe food shopping would now be better done online and we would spend our time anywhere where there were no French sticks and bottles of wine!

Life became a massive juggling act of keeping my mother safe and happy, plus trying to keep myself sane. My mother could be difficult, unreasonable, violent, and quite simply wanted to live her own life, with absolutely no insight into her own cognitive or physical impairments. She would cancel the carers and say I was taking her out, meaning she would have no lunch. She would try and make drinks with gravy and tap water, quite often spilling it and then slipping on the wood floor, ambulances would be called, and the constant stress and pressure just never ended.

We discovered the GP had stopped her blood pressure tablets a few months before the brain haemorrhage. She was supposed to go back and get a different prescription, but she never did. She had been a ticking time bomb all along and we didn't know as she was a very private person in many ways. As her condition deteriorated, they increased her care visits to four a day, but the camera became a double-edged sword as I watched her combing her hair with the remote control, gesturing passionately into thin air, or pretending she was smoking.

I developed a routine to try and help me cope. I'd get up, check my mother was ok on the camera, and then do my own housework before going to sit with her before doing her housework and chores. After lunch, I'd drive to the nearby quay and just sit and take in the silence, praying for a miracle that would bring our mother back to us. The worse thing in many ways was that physically, she now wasn't too bad but mentally, the brain injury had ravaged her and completely changed her personality.

The peace and tranquillity of the quayside retreat recharged me a little for the evening rota until it was time for bed. The thing I hated most was having to lock her in at night but I had no choice, as every night, she told me how she wanted to go to the dance as all her friends were waiting for her. I sometimes felt like an evil woman coming into her house and stopping her happiness, yet at other times she smiled at me with a warmth I'd forgotten existed. I drove home to my own house, usually to be greeted by a grumpy husband who resented the effect this was having on me and was angered by the complete lack of suitable placements for my mother. Being in your 70s with a brain injury didn't tick any boxes and the best fit was dementia which at that point, she didn't have.

What fresh hell is this? I thought, and how would it all end?

By 2014 I was feeling burnt out again. My mother had started to do some strange things, like taking all the pictures off the wall and stacking them in a corner or packing all her belongings in plastic carrier bags. She said she wanted to go home but no matter how many times I tried to explain this was home, she didn't believe me, saying there was another house down the road and her husband and children were waiting for her. She wanted to go back to a house that didn't exist, to my dad who had died fifteen years ago and to children now grown who were standing in front of her, but it was impossible to explain that to her. In her mind, she was forty years old. It was just heart breaking for everyone, especially her.

At the end of 2014, I saw my consultant who said I couldn't really put this surgery off much longer. The rectum was causing new problems so that needed to be checked, I was due yet another ultrasound and he told me I may as well just get the operation done so I could move on with life. The operation was scheduled for three months hence which would be January 2015. He said I'd probably be in hospital about a week. In some ways, I saw this as a way to break the cycle we were in. Without my input, maybe my mother would get more appropriate care and maybe for once I could relax about my health knowing all the badness had finally gone, giving me the strength and ability to concentrate more on my mother in her final years.

How wrong could I have been!

CHAPTER 3

Christmas 2014 came and went, and the prospect of the surgery weighed heavily on my mind. I'd been having counselling since the summer of 2014 as I'd had difficulty dealing with life and in particular, my poor mother's situation. My marriage was also groaning at the seams because of the relentless stress and worries. Andrew had reasonably good health and missed the life he had hoped for. But we pulled together and hoped the operation would be a turning point for us. The chronic pelvic problems would be alleviated, the suspect mass would be no more and the leaky painful rectal stump a distant memory.

As it was eighty miles from home and we had to be on the ward by 7am on the Monday, we spent the weekend prior to the operation in a nice hotel near the hospital. We had a great weekend, I felt well and we enjoyed each other's company which was very welcome after such a long trawl of stress. My sister, daughter and her partner would, of course, take my place and my mother's sisters had agreed to help out. In any event, I'd be home soon. I'd even thought I could move in with her after my op and we could support each other. How deluded was I!

We arrived at the hospital and I was still having serious doubts, even at this late stage, but I saw my consultant and immediately felt reassured. I was admitted, signed the consent forms, and as I walked to theatre, I kissed Andrew, saying jokingly, 'See you on the other side.'

I'd had so many operations over the years, the time in the anaesthetic room held no fears for me. The monitors were attached, the obligatory chats with the staff, me apologising for my short-sightedness as my glasses were taken away, the talk of the relaxant that would make me feel like I'd had a few too many wines – this was routine to me. Then the words 'sharp scratch' were uttered, which meant I would soon have the big phial of white liquid that would anaesthetise me for the 35th time and all the badness would be gone and life would begin again . . .

I awoke from the op in so much pain, I felt paralysed. I just couldn't move and as the nurse bellowed instructions about the morphine pump, I struggled to take it all in. I don't remember much other than one of the consultants telling me he hadn't managed to remove the rectum, and the other one later saying it had been difficult but they managed to do the hysterectomy. I went back to the ward where Andrew was waiting. I'd been having surgery almost annually for thirty-two of the thirty-four years we had been married. He was always there waiting, reading his book or more recently Kindle, secretly hoping that maybe this would be the last time. We used to dream of doing normal things, like going on a cruise or a long-haul flight. He wanted to show me the wonderful places he'd been to, places I'd been denied owing to my health. I can't say I ever felt I missed out on these things as, to me, a good year was a year without surgery. But still we had dreams and maybe we would now be able to realise some of them before it was too late! After all, the menopause was to be my panacea and with my ovaries gone, this was now a reasonable prospect, wasn't it?

He held my hand and I drifted in and out of sleep which was a welcome break from the extreme pain I was in. He must have gone back to the hotel at some point and the next thing I remember was my consultant checking my catheter bag, saying it was all looking good. He had a big coat on, it was January, and I remember thinking 'please don't go.' I felt as if I was in another world, everything looked totally surreal and it was if I was living out my life in some kind of slow motion.

Andrew came and sat with me all day. I remember I'd brought some nice toiletries in but when the nurses encouraged me to move and wash, I would have been more capable of eating my feet. I just couldn't function. I felt I wanted to somehow crawl inside the bed, I was restless, I felt very, very strange. They said it was the after effects of the surgery or the anaesthetic or the drugs wearing off, all perfectly normal and nothing to worry about. They gave me Buscopan to ease my increasing abdominal spasms and they then tried to feed me chicken soup which made me heave.

On the evening of Day Two, a new nurse came on duty and Andrew knew her dad from the police. Glad to see a friendly face, they chatted and he expressed his concern at how sleepy I was and how he'd never seen me like this before. She listened intently and kindly encouraged me to get up and try and walk around the bed. I would feel better, she urged, and it may get my stoma working. It's quite usual for your gut to go into 'sulk' mode after abdominal surgery. The medical name is ileus whereby your gut just stops working. It's extremely painful but usually resolves itself in time. Until it does start working, you feel like death would be the better option.

I eased myself out of the bed with help and stood up. I felt like I was going to pass out. In all the years of surgery, this was a whole new experience. I felt like I'd woken up in a different body. I took a few steps with Andrew's help and everyone encouraged me, telling me how well I was doing. I stared at them through glassy eyes and tried to smile my thanks. I suddenly felt a warm feeling on my left leg. I gestured to Andrew who lifted my gown and noticed the drain bag to the left was full and leaking, leaving a greenish puddle at my feet. The nurse guided me back to bed rather quickly. She fiddled with the bag and mumbled it looked like bile. Now, despite having a reasonable insight into my health and surgery in general, this meant nothing to me or my husband. She called a doctor and the next thing I knew, my gynaecologist appeared. It was 9.30 at night, this did not bode well. They explained it was looking as if my bowel had perforated, and what was coming into the bag was bowel contents which were now swilling around in my pelvic cavity. I needed IV antibiotics immediately, but I also needed to be transferred to the City Hospital where they were more equipped to deal with this type of emergency. I felt completely terrified as I looked at my poor husband who was speechless and in tears.

The ambulance arrived and I was transferred from bed to trolley. The paramedics looked young and healthy and how I envied them their exuberance. One of them was joking how if there was a bed for me at City Hospital, it would be a miracle. Andrew asked what he meant and he just joked, 'You'll soon find out.' Andrew explained that the consultant had phoned in advance to make the arrangements, but he said nothing, just smirked. He irritated me intensely and I prayed he was wrong.

The nurse came with us on the short journey and Andrew followed in the car, having quickly gathered up all my belongings. This was the same hospital my mother had gone to, following her brain haemorrhage. The vastness of it still frightened me, it all frightened me.

We arrived in A&E to chaos, people everywhere, trolleys backed up and no one had a clue who I was, despite the nurse's remonstrations. She phoned the hospital I'd come from and there was even talk of me going back there as there really was 'no room at the inn'. I could feel myself drifting in and out of consciousness as Andrew looked on, still holding my hand.

The next thing I remember is being on a ward, with a cannula inserted into my hand and several bags of liquid being put up. I lay there, not knowing what was happening. It was midnight and Andrew looked a broken man as I held his hand more tightly than ever before. I begged them to let him sleep in the chair next to me, but they said no visitors allowed overnight. He had no option but to sleep in the car in the car park on a freezing January night.

The stomach cramps were getting worse and then suddenly I felt a gush and was aware of a warm sticky feeling between my legs. My stomach turned as I thought I was bleeding to death. With every spasm of my gut, a pool of liquid gushed out and it seemed to be coming from my vagina. I couldn't reach the bell or cry out, so I raised my hand and the lady opposite rang the bell for me. Two nurses came, very young and I think of Philippine origin, they spoke poor English. I told them I was bleeding and as they lifted the sheet and moved my gown, they mumbled something to each other. Off they went and came back with lots of large pads and proceeded to mop up the puddles of liquid between my legs. As they now had the torch on me, I could see it wasn't actually blood but the green liquid I now knew to be bile. My bowel contents were flooding out of me vaginally! This was pure hell; how could this even happen? I wanted Andrew but they said no, but they would call a doctor. Doctors came and went but as my observations were reasonably stable, they wanted to wait until morning. My colorectal consultant's name was mentioned over and over, but it seemed he was out of town and would not be back until mid-morning. Nothing would or could be done until then, unless, of course, I deteriorated further.

I spent the night in a morphine-induced haze. Every time I shut my eyes, I felt as if I was being transported at great speed down a narrow tunnel. Always before I reached the end of the tunnel, I woke up with a massive feeling of terror inside, making me too afraid to close my eyes again. Hallucinations of massive spiders chased me around the room, making me think I'd died and gone to hell. I heard a spine-chilling scream and then realised it was me! That turned out to be the longest and most terrifying night of my life and the start of a seemingly never-ending nightmare.

CHAPTER 4

The next few days were a blur of doctors and scans as well as endless blood tests and monitoring. My consultant had returned and confirmed my bowel had indeed perforated. Worryingly, he looked concerned which was unusual for him. He didn't really know why but the area of the repeated aspirations for the endometriotic cysts had welded itself to my bowel and womb. The operation had become very difficult and they had to abandon attempts to remove the rectal stump as I had lost a lot of blood. Annie and her partner were now with me and asked if the perforation could be repaired. We were told it was too dangerous, the area was very friable and wouldn't stand up to further surgery. He explained I would go back to theatre that day to have a more substantive drainage tube inserted deep into my pelvis, which would be brought outside through my abdominal wall and the output would drain into a bag. I would not be able to eat or drink and I would be fed through my central vein. If it were going to heal, it would do so within three months.

I just couldn't take it all in. I never realised this was even possible. I'd never had any complications before and now it seemed my surgical 'luck' had well and truly run out. I was heartbroken. I held Annie's hand and just wished and prayed I could turn the clock back. Of course, all of this was made so much worse for me because I'd been warned to avoid invasive surgery unless my life was at risk but now it was too late. We were all in a state of absolute shock and disbelief at this terrible outcome to what was supposed to be a routine surgery.

Annie and her partner returned home as they had jobs to go to and of course, my mother to look after, as my sister was trying to cope alone. Andrew found accommodation in the form of a bedsit fairly near the hospital. As it was January, he had it at a cheaper rate which helped as we had not planned on this. His business - he had recently become a self-employed electrician - was in its infancy but it had to take a back seat and he passed on his scheduled work to colleagues.

We tried to remain positive but it was very difficult. The hospital had strict visiting times with no discretion, as every case on the ward seemed to be serious. I saw things I never knew existed, like the lady with a bag on her neck who used to spit all day long. She was unable to eat or drink and was fed through a tube in her stomach. She explained her oesophagus had collapsed in on itself, meaning food would not go down and it was too dangerous to operate. She had come in to have it dilated and if this was successful, she could eat Quavers and drink some water, that was it. I used to watch her putting on her make up and painting her nails, saying it was important to her to look the best she could, despite the bag in her neck and what she had to deal with every day. Her courage was humbling. I could not imagine living like that, yet she had been like it for several years. The lady in the bed next to me had come in to have her gall bladder removed but had developed complications – she had been in hospital for seven months, she had young children and said her life was in tatters. As I listened to their stories, I could feel my mental health deteriorating as the magnitude of what had happened to me sunk in.

As the days passed with no improvement, the staff said I would be moved to another ward where I would be given an intravenous feed. I hadn't eaten or drunk anything for eleven days and despite being on saline drips to keep me hydrated, I had a thirst that is impossible to comprehend. My mouth was so dry I couldn't speak and the spray they gave me made me gag. What was worse was that no one acknowledged my fears. Why couldn't someone just say the truth and acknowledge the seriousness of my situation? But I was silenced and under pressure to pretend I was coping mentally when I quite clearly was not. I felt if one more person told me to be positive, I would scream. I just wanted someone to validate my emotional experience, not play it down. This outcome was bad and there was no denying it!

I was taken to ultrasound where they inserted a line into the central vein next to my heart. This was seriously scary, and I felt I was plunging deeper into absolute despair. They said the line was called a Broviac line and it could be left in for several months which just distressed me even more. That night, I was hooked up to a machine and began to receive my Total Parenteral Nutrition (TPN). This is a method of feeding that bypasses the gastrointestinal tract. Fluids are given into a vein to provide most of the nutrients the body needs but, like everything, there are various side effects and risks which I just didn't want to know about. Thanks to the IV fluids and lack of movement, I had ballooned to sixteen stone! I was told that, once the TPN started nourishing me and I could move about a bit, I would start to feel better.

Being on TPN meant more frequent monitoring by the nurses, while your body adapted to it. There were a few people on the ward on TPN and I would see them walking around, pushing their trolleys hooked up to bags of the fluid that was keeping them alive. Apparently, they were encouraged to do laps of the ward, as movement was good and sitting in bed was not. I spoke to some of them and they told me their stories which ranged from serious Crohn's disease, whereby they had lost most of their bowel, to blood clots that had destroyed much of their bowel, to a bowel blockage. The reasons were many and while none of the recipients wanted to be on TPN, it was a life-or-death situation. Without it, they would literally starve to death. Despite having had bowel issues for most of my adult life, plus of course having a stoma when I was in my twenties, I always had a good appetite, a love of chocolate and red wine. I had always struggled to lose weight, now I was faced with a gut that may never work properly again. To add to it all, every time I walked even a short distance, ominous-looking liquid came out from 'down below'. Now that certainly was some new kind of hell and I was not coping at all.

I asked the nurse to tell me how common it was for a bowel to perforate and not be repaired. I was worried that I'd become very ill with this leak in my bowel. It was during this conversation that the word 'fistula' first reared its ugly head. She said the body was very clever and would form an abnormal connection called a fistula which would hopefully stop me getting sepsis. She said they were one of the risks of surgery, especially with a 'history like mine'. I was learning not to ask questions if I couldn't take the answers. When she left, of course I turned to Dr Google to learn some more – certainly the wrong thing to do! To my horror, I read:

The development of a Gastrointestinal fistula is a catastrophic complication of a surgical procedure in the vicinity of the abdominal cavity. Patients continue to die from fistulas, and the cause of death is nearly always infection.

A fistula is an abnormal connection between an organ, vessel, or intestine and another organ, vessel or intestine, or the skin. Fistulas can be thought of as tubes connecting internal tubular structures, such as arteries, veins, or intestine, to one another or to the skin. Fistulas are usually the result of trauma or surgery but can also result from infection or inflammation.

Fistula tracts must be treated because they will not heal on their own. There is a risk of developing cancer in the fistula tract if left untreated for a long period of time.

A fistula may cause complications. In some cases, fistulas might not heal and become chronic. Other potential complications include fistula drainage, sepsis, and perforation and peritonitis. Sepsis is a life-threatening illness that results from the body's response to a bacterial infection.

And so on . . .

I could find nothing positive about this newly acquired monster I had within me. I struggled to find a sympathetic nurse to talk to but of course, they had seen it all before and I was just another patient with another problem. I decided not to tell my family what I had been told as I thought it best we ask the consultant directly as Dr Google did not paint a very good picture at all.

This didn't stop me looking online to see if there were any forums dealing with this complication. I found one called Enterocutaneous Fistula Support Group, perfect or so I thought – there were just fifty-six members in the whole world! I was obviously part of a very exclusive group that no one wanted to be part of. I read three horror stories and decided to leave, it was just too traumatic. Considering just a few days ago, I'd never even heard of a fistula, it seemed there are many types and all equally awful. I found another group called Abscess and Fistula Support for Women which had thousands of members - I read their posts with tears in my eyes. Tales of repeated failed surgeries and shattered dreams seemed to be the main theme, occasionally peppered with a success story of someone who had healed. I reminded myself how people only tend to visit such forums if they have ongoing problems and not if they had healed and were getting on with life. I decided not to participate in either group for now but would re visit when I was cured and maybe offer some hope to someone going through what I was going through.

CHAPTER 5

My consultant confirmed I did indeed have a fistula with tracks into the vagina. The best way to treat this, was, as he had already explained - nil by mouth, continue on TPN, watch, wait and hope. As I was making such slow progress, my hospital stay seemed never-ending as the days grew into weeks and weeks into months.

After about six weeks, the output from the drainage tube had reduced slightly as had the vaginal output. They said I could have sips of water which progressed to cups of tea to morsels of food. But the TPN continued as I was unable to eat enough to nourish me without the output from the drainage tube increasing. Every sip was measured, as was everything I passed in the form of urine plus output from the drainage and stoma bags. It was excruciating as the whole focus of my life was this fluid chart to help identify any deficits. Half the time I wasn't sure they were even completing them properly and this just stressed me out even more.

A fistula is classified as low, medium or high output, depending on the amount it exudes. The higher up the bowel it is, the higher the output. If the output is higher than 1 litre per day, it is likely you will have to remain on TPN to ensure adequate nutrition is received. My output was low to medium which was still too much for my liking. I wanted it to be zero, I wanted it gone. I just couldn't accept it and hated what it had done to my life. I should say our life as Andrew and my family were just as devastated.

I became fixated on it all and was constantly checking the bag in the vain hope it would be empty. If I did have a good day and it was empty, I'd be ecstatic, only to come crashing down the next day when it invariably filled again. It just wasn't healing quickly enough and I knew that if it didn't heal within three months, then it probably was never going to, although opinions on that one varied. The thought of going home on TPN terrified me. I couldn't imagine a life without food and drink - going for coffee, a nice meal with a glass or two of wine - it was all as automatic as breathing.

As I wandered the corridors day in and day out, I realised I had to somehow find the resilience to get me through this. But telling myself this didn't help at all as depression was really taking hold. I just couldn't see the point in anything anymore and started to have really black thoughts. The doctors would tell me how important it was to be positive and how a negative outlook reduced my chances of recovering, but this only made me feel worse, as if I somehow chose to be depressed. I didn't seem to have any control of my runaway toxic mind.

One day, I got talking to another patient in the corridor. He was about my age but looked really unwell. He had a yellowish pallor and was very thin. He told me how he'd come in to have a cyst on his liver removed but developed complications and ended up losing quite a large amount of his liver, plus the cyst turned out to be malignant. He would be starting chemotherapy once he was a little stronger.

I broke down as I listened to his harrowing story and told him how hopeless I was and even though I wasn't going through anything like his story, I just couldn't accept what had happened. I asked him how he remained so strong and focused. 'What choice do I have?' he asked. A good question as of course he didn't have any choice, it was sink or swim and he intended to swim for as long as he could. He was a new grandad and he wanted to see his granddaughter grow up. He told me I was probably in shock and in a way, losing your health was a form of grief.

I had never really thought about it in that context but it certainly resonated with me. Grief is after all an emotional response to loss and I had lost something very precious, my health. Finally, someone was validating my feelings and allowing me to be sad about the outcome I'd had to surgery. He was so thoughtful, despite going through his own nightmare. He wished me well and we went off to our respective wards. I never saw him again but I never forgot his kindness and empathy.

The days were long but thankfully there was a good internet connection which proved to be my lifeline. I could talk to my family on messenger and we decided to scale the visits down to three times a week. It was too stressful making the 180-mile round trip daily, apart from the financial cost which was a major consideration.

I started writing a blog and chatting to people online. I was still avoiding any sites to do with fistula as they were all extremely depressing and I soon stopped writing the blog too - I really needed hope but wasn't finding it online. I just wasn't healing and was very fearful at what lay ahead.

But one forum really helped. It was a menopause forum and I had been a member since 2010 when I started on the menopause road. Ironically, I hadn't really suffered half the problems some forum members had but it became a massive help to me and possibly saved my sanity on more than one occasion.

Prior to my operation, I spoke to them about my fears of having the surgery, wanting their opinions on it. In 2014, the year before the op, I asked them about my medical dilemma:

October 2014 - Hi ladies, I went to see the bowel surgeon last week as I feel this dilemma is taking its toll. I have become depressed and to be honest, impossible to live with. As you all know, the situation is I need preventative surgery - I have longstanding Crohn's in my bottom which is an increased cancer risk plus I have longstanding gynae probs which have left lots of scars and question marks as to what is going on inside. Every test I have results in more questions and queries. I can't seem to live with the thought of doing nothing and hope nothing nasty develops but I am equally terrified of the surgery. But having spoken to the surgeon last week he feels I need to get this done - he said it may never become a serious problem but if it did, because of my history, they may not be able to remove it. So I've decided to go ahead with the surgery, it will be a few months yet but my decision is made.

Lots of replies and comments followed, mostly encouraging me and pleased I had finally made this very difficult decision:

'Sometimes we must take a leap of faith and let the medical profession make the decisions. I am pleased you have reached this point and seem positive about what lays (sic) ahead.'

'To me, the definition of bravery is doing the things you are terrified of doing. You are certainly a heroine in my books! Keep posting and whenever you feel down and scared. We are here for you. X'

*'I know you must have deep reservations about this surgery, who wouldn't! But the decision is made, you trust these top doctors so get it done and move on with your life. Just remember once this is over to take all the time **you** need to recover. This is your time now.'*

On 24 January, I had to tell them the bad news that things hadn't gone to plan:

Hi Ladies, I had the op and it developed a nasty complication. Basically, my small bowel was so adhered to my womb etc that it was damaged during the surgery. No one expected this outcome obviously, I've been unlucky they said. Long story short but my bowel contents started leaking into my pelvic cavity and I became seriously ill. I am now physically better but my gut is not working, in this scenario it can take months to heal as sometimes more surgery is not possible as it will make things much worse.

I am devastated. I am in a massive hospital - a specialised unit 80 miles from home. I am not in any great pain thank God - I can't eat or drink - just ice cubes. I am being nourished by a special parenteral nutrition which goes into a vein by my heart. I'm really afraid, ladies. The plan is to completely rest the bowel for it to heal. If it heals, which could take months, they may then start me eating. If it doesn't heal it would be more surgery or I will return home being vein fed which I cannot accept.

I can't deal with it. It's definitely one day at a time stuff but my mind is excellent at the 'what if' game. I'm trying to develop new pastimes as in effect this is my life for a while. Andrew and daughter are heartbroken. My mother is coping ok with carers for now - the rest of the family pulling together, my sister and the twins are ok. All the time I have spent on here bleating on about rubbish I so wish I could turn the clock back.

Has anyone been in this type of life changing scenario and can anyone provide any help on positive thinking or how to adopt a one day at a time mentality? Thanks ladies x

The thread ran for 250 pages and was read nearly 40,000 times. They truly were my guardian angels and helped me through the long, dark days.

41

Two months into my stay, the output from the tube had decreased to the point where it was decided I should now start to eat whilst they weaned me off the TPN. They said there were no guarantees of success and the only way of knowing was to try eating. If I became ill, then the TPN would continue.

Eating became a source of great anxiety but staying on TPN seemed like a fate almost worse than death. I started off with some apple juice and a piece of toast for breakfast, a yogurt for lunch and some cheese and biscuits for dinner. Coupled with the protein drinks, this provided enough calories to sustain me. I was weaned off the TPN but the line was kept in 'just in case'. Deep down, I didn't feel confident but I was so desperate to go home, I never displayed my fears and, in any event, I knew no one would listen. I'd been branded as anxious and if ever I seemed down or upset about something, it was put down to my 'extreme anxiety'. I did wonder how other people would feel in this situation. Was it just me or were my reactions normal? I'd come into hospital relatively well with a full and reasonably active life back home (plus a brain-damaged mother who needed me), and was now this – a broken human being, wracked with anxiety over a damaged gut, poo coming out of my lady bits – who wouldn't be anxious?

The psychiatric team had put my anxiety down to a 'bad inpatient experience' and said it would get better when I regained my health. This was no help at all, they were missing the point entirely as there were no guarantees I would regain my health. A fistula is a massive challenge for doctors and patients and as many of my fellow patients told me, can lead to a life of constant hospital admissions and chronic health problems. Emotionally, I was in a very, very bad place. One of my most precious possessions – my health – had been taken away but I just had to accept it, and I wasn't even allowed to react to it as it upset people. I had to bury my emotions to stop other people feeling uncomfortable, at least that seemed to be the deal. It felt like a pretty raw one for me.

However, I discovered meditation which was a great help. On one of their many visits, Annie and her partner downloaded several meditation apps and bought me some really nice headphones. Whenever I found my head becoming overwhelmed by black thoughts, I donned my headphones and relaxed into a world of tranquillity, where, for at least a short while, I could escape the trauma in my mind.

I was discharged at the end of March 2015, totally off TPN and as far I was concerned, on the road to recovery. The latest scan had suggested an improving picture and the gynaecologist who had carried out the hysterectomy was delighted to tell me the histology from the hysterectomy confirmed no malignancies were found. Whilst I was obviously relieved to hear that, it didn't take away the enormity of what had happened but I truly believed my nightmare was coming to an end. The fistula was finally healing and would hopefully soon be a distant memory.

CHAPTER 6

Being home after three months in hospital was strange. I felt somehow as if I didn't belong and remember getting very upset when Andrew had moved the toaster to the other side of the kitchen. The house had always been my domain. I was a bit of a neat freak and it was a bone of contention between us. I called our three cats and they all looked at me with disdain, as if to say, 'And where have you been?' The house looked drab and unloved. I spotted a lonely Christmas decoration lurking in the corner of the lounge whilst the daffodils were flowering outside on the patio. I had left home in mid-winter and came home in spring. But it felt so good to be back – finally my recovery could begin in earnest.

Andrew wanted to get 'back to normal' as soon as possible and he returned to work a few days after I came home, which suited me as I was left to my own devices. I spent the days pottering about but was still very nervous about everything. Every visit to the loo was filled with anxiety for fear of discharge appearing on the pad, plus every pain filled me with dread in case it led to something more serious putting me back in hospital. Eating became a tortuous experience as I only felt 'safe' with the nutritional drinks I'd been prescribed. To make matters worse, my discharge from hospital coincided with big changes at my local GP surgery. My long-term GP had retired and many of the others who knew me had left, to be replaced with locum doctors.

Leaving the protective hospital environment was scary and made me realise I really wasn't that healed at all. I found myself becoming increasingly insular, cocooned in the safety net of home, not wanting to go out and mix with people and do normal things. Andrew and I would occasionally go for coffee but I was totally on edge all the time, scared to eat, constantly checking my dressings and totally scared of life. The operation going wrong had totally rocked my world and I was still reeling from the whole experience.

We had had some wonderful news, though – our daughter was pregnant! It was early days but all was good, the baby was due early 2016 and they had chosen not to know the sex which made it all the more exciting. This was a massive incentive for me to get better as I so wanted to be able to help Annie and her partner with the new baby.

My mother continued to live at her home with the help of carers, plus lots of family 'pop ins'. I'd obviously been to see her since coming out of hospital and while she seemed ok physically, I could see a massive deterioration in her cognition. She had periods of complete normality but then, almost within seconds, would become very confused and agitated.

One evening in May 2015, things reached a very low point. It was a Friday night and Annie phoned me to say she had had a phone call from the carers to say my mother was on the road, being very aggressive and refusing to go back inside. Annie and her partner went down but there was no reasoning with her, and they struggled to get her back in. The carers felt it was becoming increasingly difficult to take responsibility for her, owing to her intermittent and unpredictable bizarre behaviour and they would have to report this latest incident as a serious concern. They eventually managed to get her back to bed and we monitored her from the cameras in our respective houses to make sure she was safe. Once in bed, she invariably would sleep all night without issues.

I felt so useless as I was unable to move in with her, as I found the physical and mental demands of dealing with a brain-injured person, especially as it was my mother with whom I had a deep emotional connection, just too exhausting. Andrew was totally opposed too as he knew I would take on too much which could hinder any chance I had of recovering further. He knew the emotional distress of my mother's situation was destroying me. He also felt that the more we were doing, the less help we would get from the authorities. Things just weren't sustainable with my health taking such a downward turn.

A few days later I had another phone call from a very distressed Annie. My mother had somehow found a plastic cigarette, had managed to light it and was smoking it exuberantly whilst a small fire smouldered by her feet! Annie was in town but had noticed it on the camera which was on her phone. I rushed down as quickly I could, but as it was lunch time, the carer had beaten me to it.

I entered the hall of her small, terraced cottage with my heart in my throat. I heard the carer talking to my mother in an adjacent room, so I knew she was ok. The carer shouted, telling me to go out to the kitchen but to be careful. The kitchen looked as if blood had been smeared all over the floor and hob. My heart calmed down quickly, however, as it soon became apparent it wasn't blood after all but cherry red lipstick! My mother had managed to turn the hob on (she must have climbed onto a stool to access the electricity supply), and then proceeded to light the plastic cigarette along with several lipsticks which had melted and dripped to the floor, her footsteps leaving a blood-like trail as she walked the short distance back to her room. I went to talk to the carer who told me she would have to report this as another 'incident of concern' as she was quite clearly no longer safe to be left alone. I took hold of my mother's hand and asked her gently, 'What have you been up to then?'. She replied quite sternly, 'Will you hurry up and make dinner, Len will be home soon.' Len was my late father who had died sixteen years ago. The reality of our dire situation was becoming more evident by the day. The complexity of her brain injury was so difficult to manage that her days at home were undoubtedly numbered.

A few days later, the carers found her literally buried under a massive pile of coats and blankets, with just her head popping out the top. She had taken all the pictures off the wall and packed them neatly into carrier bags which were lined up in the passage. She told me she was going home whether I liked it or not, her husband and children were waiting.

Following this, she was hospitalised as it was thought she may have had another bleed which could explain her increasingly bizarre behaviour. She remained in hospital for three months. There were no beds locally and this hospital was a 120-mile round trip and of course, I couldn't drive. Yet more stress for everyone and more sadness at my mother's dire situation.

A few days after the fire incident, I noticed a hole had appeared on my midline scar, a tiny pinhead-sized, perfectly round, weeping hole. My stomach knotted, that now all too familiar feeling of terror engulfing me whenever even the possibility of a fistula reared its ugly head. The discharge wasn't faecal but it was yellow. Perhaps it was pus, an infection maybe. I put a dressing on it and sat on the bed and cried so hard I thought my heart would break. The traumatic events of the last few months suddenly hit me like a high-speed train.

I fell into a deep sleep, only to be awoken by Andrew a few hours later. He had remained in complete denial about the seriousness of my condition and hated coming home to find me unhappy or distressed. He preferred me to wear the 'happy mask' rather than show my true feelings to him as he just couldn't deal with it. To come home and find me in bed was unheard of and it annoyed him greatly which in turn deepened my feelings of isolation and loneliness. I showed him the hole on my stomach, the seepage now looking darker and more faecal. Sadly for him, he couldn't say this was all in my head as the evidence was staring him in the face.

It was 7pm so we went to our local A&E, Andrew angry at my inability to cope with anything, or so it seemed to him. We were eventually seen and a doctor stuck a probe in the hole which disappeared deep into my abdomen. He looked concerned but as all my observations were ok, he felt I should go home and he would write to my consultant.

And so it began.

CHAPTER 7

I was now convinced the fistula was lurking and that it was only a matter of time before I'd become seriously ill again. I didn't understand how you could have a hole in your bowel and stay alive. Normal life ceased to exist as I spent my days at home, scared to do anything, and even scared to move too much as it increased the vaginal flow. I was scared to eat anything normal as I noticed if I did eat something like meat or vegetables, the output from the hole in the abdominal wall would be worse. So I basically sat on the bed, a broken wreck, and became so depressed I didn't want to participate in life. The less I was coping with this, the more Andrew was also secretly falling apart. His way of coping with it all was to work and so he basically stayed out of my way. But of course, life goes on and I still had my beautiful pregnant daughter, my mother who was still in hospital, and those two little boys whom I loved unconditionally and who needed Aunty back to how she was. So I picked myself up and hid my fears as much as I could, whilst trying to embrace my 'new normal'.

In August 2015, the hospital said my mother was ready for discharge, as nothing more medically or surgically could be done for her. We were called to a meeting where it was decided she needed 24-hour care and if we couldn't provide it, then she would have to go into a home. She was 76 and clinically well, yet in her mind she was 40 years old and raring to get on with her life. My sister, daughter and I went to look at various residential and nursing homes in the vicinity. They were all awful and wholly unsuitable for my mother who had a brain injury, who could get better with the right stimulation and treatment. She had a lot of life left in her – I didn't want her labelled as yet another dementia patient and stuck in a home waiting to die. This was just heart-breaking! Now with something else to occupy my mind, I spent my days emailing, phoning, writing to anyone who would listen, about the lack of residential placements for brain-damaged people of my mother's age. Everyone listened but offered very little in the way of a solution. Whether she had dementia or a brain injury, the fact remained she needed 24-hour care and the only homes available were essentially EMI homes (homes for the elderly and mentally impaired).

I did have really great support and empathy from the Alzheimer's Society. They became a lifeline for me and helped me navigate this latest arduous journey. After several more weeks, we were given a veiled threat by the hospital that either we found somewhere or they would. On the basis the hospital she was in was not even local, owing to lack of beds, they forced our hand as otherwise we risked her being placed in a home sixty miles away. She was eventually placed in a residential home in the town where we lived. We knew some of the staff as they lived locally and the manager was bright and cheerful. She visited my mother in hospital and she took to her immediately. We were shown her room and made it as homely as we could, with lovely bedding and pictures, plus little memoirs from home. I knew deep down I was kidding myself as she would hate it but I just had no idea what else I could do. Short of moving in with her and providing the 24-hour care she needed, we really had no choice.

Discharge day arrived and I phoned to ensure everything was in order. I waited anxiously for a phone call from the home to say she had arrived. However, the phone call I received was from the ambulance men, asking if I could come and let them in. They had mistakenly taken her back to her home address as this was the address they had been given. The nurse accompanying her told me how her eyes had lit up and how pleased she was that I'd opened the windows ready for her homecoming. I explained the situation, but I was heartbroken for her, for all of us. Eventually, they drove off, next stop the care home. She became extremely distressed when she realised what was happening - all our efforts to make the transition as painless as possible had been totally quashed. We were told not to visit her for two weeks to give her time to 'settle'.

In January 2016, happier times finally came when Annie gave birth to the most gorgeous little girl, Cari. It wasn't an easy birth but mother and baby were doing well! I felt a sense of absolute joy for the first time in what seemed like many years. I was fortunate enough to be able to spend lots of time with them, which numbed the pain of what was going on elsewhere.

The discharge down below continued and another hole had opened up on my abdomen, and I was relying on dressings to keep me dry. I was still back and fore to see the colorectal surgeon but as I was clinically ok, he felt I was doing fine and just needed to get on with things. The more my consultant said, 'You're fine', the more Andrew and I bickered as my fears fell on deaf ears. By his own admission, he was very short on empathy. We were becoming more and more emotionally detached. We argued almost daily, with him reminding me I should be grateful I wasn't still being vein-fed or dead. Of course, I absolutely agreed with that but the sadness that engulfed my every waking moment was somehow stopping me from moving forward, as was the crushing realisation it was getting worse, not better, but no one, absolutely no one, seemed to believe me or acknowledge how bad this was, for fear of upsetting me.

I became afraid to express my own fears as they affected Andrew so negatively, so I buried my own feelings so he could keep his anxiety in the shadows. The consultant had said on our last visit that the fistula may not heal now but he could not say if this was as bad as it was going to get. When I asked questions about how these things progressed, he said everyone was different which at the time, didn't help! I needed some idea of what was likely to happen as time went on. When I professed my fears about gut 'exploding' and perforating again, he said there was no evidence to support that thought. It all seemed so straightforward to everyone but me and my manic mind.

My daily routine was built around the dressings and stoma bag and as much as I hated it all, it was reasonably manageable, providing I only ate cake or sandwiches and sat on the bed all day which, as you can imagine, is another recipe for disaster – hello, weight problems!

Changing the fistula bag took hours. It's not like a stoma where the bag can be changed in a few minutes. This was a long-drawn-out process whereby the skin had to be first scrupulously cleaned, then left to dry. Barrier rings and pastes had to be applied to the skin around the fistula to fill any gaps (a stomach that's had multiple surgeries is not flat and the fistula is embedded in my mid line scar) and then finally the fistula bag carefully placed *in situ*. To increase the chances of it sticking, I would then have to lie perfectly still for about forty minutes with a hot water bottle on my stomach (the heat helped the bag stick). Even after all of this, there were no guarantees as to how long it would last, could be a few hours or a few days. What I did know was if I moved around after the application of the bag, it would not last very long which is why the bags are best changed at night just before bed.

I just felt so sad about the events of the last few years and yet I didn't seem to have the emotional or physical strength to change things. I needed to lose weight and get fit but I felt so exhausted all the time. In any case, movement and good healthy food increased the discharge which traumatised me so I felt stuck on a downward spiral.

But life goes on and I had people in my life who needed me and so I had to try and somehow deal with this. Sometimes, I'd have a stern conversation with myself – telling myself that most of the darkest fears in my head had not actually materialised. My gut hadn't exploded again, the discharge down below was a bit better, I could actually turn over in bed now without excruciating pain. I could eat and drink, albeit a bit weirdly (I ate beetroot once and locked myself in the bathroom gripped with a sense of fear and dread – why, you may ask? Because beetroot is red and if anything red came out of that hole on my stomach wall, then it would prove it was a fistula). But despite me trying to convince myself this really wasn't that bad and could be so much worse, the monster within me was in control and it felt like it was leeching my strength from me.

I was still in regular contact with the ladies on the menopause forum. I'd 'chat' to them daily and I found their seemingly unending supply of support heartwarming, to say the least. When I felt Andrew could take no more of my 'moaning' as he called it, I would turn to them for support or just a chat. My husband, the fixer, just couldn't seem to connect anymore and we drifted further and further apart. Sometimes you just want someone to listen, to be there. I wanted someone to be my 'armbands' and to carry me through this awful time, just as I had always been there for everyone else.

The ladies often reminded me that, apart from the catastrophic bowel injury, I'd also had my ovaries ripped out (yes, I felt truly mutilated by this operation). But as I explained to them, no one seemed to care about that, it just didn't seem to matter. The surgical menopause I'd endured was after all 'the least of my worries'. Numerous doctors repeatedly told me how lucky I was to survive a bowel perforation and so all these 'minor problems' were to be expected. Except I didn't consider them minor. To me, they were life-changing and yet any form of acceptance was seemingly impossible. My light had most definitely gone out.

Chapter 8

In the spring of 2016, we decided to go away for a few days. My daughter, her partner and the baby would join us and we also took my beloved twin nephews. We had decided to go to the West Midlands Safari Park and stay in a nice hotel. It would be a fun thing to do for everyone and a much-needed change of focus for me.

It was quite a long journey and the first one I'd made where the destination wasn't a hospital. I had booked a VIP Safari Tour in a ranger-driven jeep as a surprise and I was looking forward to it. We arrived at the park and met the ranger at the designated meeting point. We climbed into the jeep and started our journey, starting at the Rhino House and finishing at the Meerkat Park, stopping for a light lunch at mid-day. The tour went well, and we all enjoyed it. We had the rest of the afternoon to spend at the park, but I took a back seat, preferring to sit and watch baby Cari sleeping whilst the others explored the monkey house. In the evening we booked into our hotel and then there was the dreaded evening meal. Eating was still a source of great stress to me, especially when in company. I was ravenous having barely eaten all day, yet I knew only too well what the trade-off was – eat a meal and the fistula would spring into action. I settled for a toasted sandwich whilst everyone else tucked into steak.

But all in all, my first trip out had gone well and more importantly I'd survived outside of my comfort zone, something a year ago I really didn't think was possible. Nothing bad had happened and we had fun.

A few days after we got back, I started to have some bowel spasms, the old familiar and much feared pain of a possible obstruction. A feeling of absolute dread gripped me as I tried to ignore it. I stopped eating and drank copious amounts of water to try and flush things through. I took my dressings off and my midline holes looked red. Something bad was happening and once again, I retracted into my shell. I couldn't share this with anyone as they were all feeling relaxed after our little holiday and I didn't want to spoil that.

After a few hours of agonising spasms, Andrew noticed something was wrong and said we should go to hospital. The thought of having to explain the whole saga to new doctors just devastated but off we went and after several hours, I was admitted. I was taken for a CT scan and spent an agonising night of bowel spasms and extreme nausea. My stoma had started to work a little and so I thought the worst was over.

The next morning, I felt like I'd been kicked in the stomach by an ox. I removed my dressings and there it was. The fistula had finally emerged and goodness me, it was ugly. My heart sank to my boots, and I felt sick with disappointment and disbelief that my worst fears had materialised. The pin-sized holes had merged and this hole was about the size of a ten pence piece. It was bright red on the outside and the inside was like a bubbling volcano spitting out poo and blood. It was grotesque.

The on-call consultant come round and was quite blunt, telling me I had a fistula and I had to manage it, no operation would fix it and I was lucky it wasn't worse! He was very harsh and despite me saying there'd been no evidence of a fistula on my previous scans and I'd been told it was a sinus hole and would heal, he was not convinced. He explained in a very blunt manner that if it doesn't heal within about three months, it would never heal, it was physiologically impossible. He stressed, in no uncertain terms, that I needed to get used to it as no one would operate on me again unless my life was at risk. Off he walked, leaving me a babbling wreck. My own consultant from City Hospital is such a lovely man with a way of saying things that somehow made me feel reassured, but this guy well and truly failed the 'bedside manner' test.

As it was a weekend, there were no stoma nurses on duty and I was told I had to manage it until Monday when I could see someone. I felt terrible - hungry yet now terrified to eat for fear of what would happen. I was discharged and told I would receive a follow up appointment in due course. That was that. I'd prayed for sixteen months for it not to be a fistula and here it was.

I felt broken all over again as I spent the weekend dabbing poo that was seeping out of my abdominal wall. The bags just wouldn't stick as my skin was so excoriated. I was readmitted to hospital the next day when I developed a high fever and was then transferred to the City Hospital where I remained for six weeks. I had sepsis so was quickly administered intravenous antibiotics by the bucketful. Then followed a visit from the stoma nurses who helped me find a bag for the fistula that didn't leak. Having had my ileostomy for so long, the management of a fistula was a very different beast. It was recessed, on my midline scar which lay in a valley on my butchered stomach. My worst nightmare was unfolding before my eyes. The fistula monster had well and truly made his presence known.

So, reality had hit. My hopes of it not being a fistula dashed, I had to find a way of dealing with this. Annie would be returning to work soon and she needed me to help with the baby. In all the years of my health problems, nothing had come close to the way this affected me. I think it was because never in my wildest nightmares did I expect this outcome to that hysterectomy which I was told 'would be difficult but doable'. I'd never had any serious complications in all the years of surgery and the one operation that was supposed to take away doubt about 'the suspect mass' had actually nearly destroyed me, with the ripple effect on my closest family devastating. They all watched me go from a confident, capable person to a quiet, joyless mess gripped with anxiety and regret. Something had to change, I was sinking fast.

I tried various things to promote healing and read a lot about nutrition. The problem was the foods needed to heal our bodies were the foods that caused me, or rather my fistula, problems. Even though I now knew it was a fistula, I still couldn't deal with the leakage, especially if something identifiable came out, like a seed or a piece of lettuce - that would send me into a tailspin. Stupid, I know, but the constant reminder I had a hole in my bowel held the same terror for me then as it had eighteen months earlier when this nightmare began. I tried reflexology which was lovely but made no difference. I even tried a healer who was a three-hour round trip away but again no change. My poor husband was very sceptical about this, yet he sat in the car for hours on end, hoping I'd found something that gave me hope or at least made me smile. Plus of course a fistula is a massive trickster! Some weeks it would get better, and I'd think it was healing! The hole would reduce in size, discharge would reduce and I would feel quite well. I would wake up and be pain free and think the nightmare was over. But of course, within a few days, my world would be shattered again as the hole reopened and it all came crashing down. I was back to square one again.

I continued to see my consultant regularly and he remained his usual positive self. I always felt better for seeing him. Even if he could not actually do anything, he had the ability to say the right things. I felt safe with him around. I genuinely believed this was a temporary disaster and normal life would resume. I asked about a possible repair to the fistula and he said it wasn't impossible but I would have to wait two years to ensure everything was totally healed and any scar tissue had softened.

So that became my aim, to get as fit as possible and count down the days until the monster could be eradicated.

Chapter 9

The date was set for 4th March 2017, the day I would be repaired, and the fistula gone. The last few months had been tough, with repeated infections requiring antibiotics and painkillers just to get through the days.

The day of the surgery arrived. We had to phone in the morning to check there was a bed. This in itself was frustrating as they couldn't say and told me to ring back at 3pm. The hospital was a three-hour round trip and Andrew and I lay on the bed waiting for 3 o'clock to arrive so we could phone again. At one point, we even said we would cancel it all, the antibiotics were helping, and I felt ok. My beautiful little granddaughter was now fourteen months old and we had got into a routine of looking after her, along with the twins who came to 'Aunty's Diner' every day for their tea, followed by pancakes. I couldn't bear the thought of saying goodbye to my family but realised we had to get this done for me to have any kind of a normal life again. I rang the hospital as instructed and we were told there was a bed so off we set with a very heavy heart. We arrived at the ward, where everyone was busy, so we sat for a while and eventually I was taken to my bed. Andrew had again booked a hotel to save the travelling and we said our goodbyes and off he went. That night, I was given special drinks to aid recovery and feeling reasonably ok, was so looking forward to being fistula-free.

Saturday 4th March 2017

The morning of 4th March dawned, and my consultant came in to deal with the formalities. Having read so much about fistulas and the exceedingly difficult job of repairing them, I was very nervous and signed the consent form with great trepidation. I'd never given this part of the process much thought before but now everything traumatised me. Andrew came to the ward and we kissed goodbye as I was wheeled to theatre.

I returned to the ward about six hours later. The consultant had told Andrew the surgery had been more difficult than he had anticipated. It had been necessary to make three joins in the bowel and he'd had to dissect part of my bladder. This sounded very worrying as the more joins, the more chances of one of them failing but I felt ok, the usual post-op pain treated with morphine, and I went to sleep feeling optimistic. The best news was my stoma bag had started to work which was an excellent sign. I messaged everyone back home the good news.

Sunday 5th March 2017

The next morning, I awoke and didn't feel great. Again, I was assured it was all down to post-operative pain and I would have to be patient. Andrew visited at lunchtime, and it was then we noticed the drainage bag to my left was full. My heart sank. I felt as if I was going to pass out as I knew what this meant. We called the nurse who confirmed it looked as if a leak had developed in the bowel again. The consultant was called and I went back to theatre.

It was a Sunday afternoon and theatre was quiet. The anaesthetist was from my part of the world, and we chatted as he put me off to sleep, telling me, as they do, to 'Think of something nice'. I cannot remember what I was thinking but remember feeling immensely sad and worried. Why had my bowel leaked again? The consultant said I'd been unlucky but he said that last time . . .?

I came back from theatre many hours later and by now, Andrew had stopped asking the medical staff questions. He was so worn out and just could not deal with it all. There were no guarantees here, this was yet more major surgery but hopefully it would be fine. That word again – 'fine' – every time they said it would be fine, it was anything but.

Tuesday 7th March 2017

I awoke feeling awful, worse than awful, no words could explain how bad I felt. I could barely move for pain and overwhelming nausea. I had a tube in my nose, a nasogastric tube which must have been put in in theatre. Attached to this was a bag which was full to bursting of a dark glossy green liquid which had a distinctive sickly smell. I patted my stomach and could feel my stoma bag was completely empty, this was bad news. The dreaded ileus had struck whereby your gut stops working, hopefully temporarily. The painful lack of movement means that, apart from extreme nausea and a feeling you are going to explode, the bile produced by your digestive system has nowhere to go and backs up. I felt as if I was choking on my own bodily fluids, yet the thirst I was experiencing was just torture.

Andrew came and we sat whilst I drifted in and out of sleep. He bathed my lips with a wet cloth, and I had a sneaky dribble of water which was just not enough. There was so much I wanted to tell him but I had no strength and besides which, I didn't want to upset him further. I could see by his face that he was really struggling. My consultant came and looked at my charts and said I was doing ok. I did not feel ok, I wanted to go to sleep and never wake up. I wanted to phone Annie to tell her how much I loved her. I wanted to tell her I couldn't do this anymore, but she had to promise me she would carry on being the beautiful person she was, the best daughter ever and the most wonderful mother to Cari. She was the best thing I has achieved in my life and all my proudest and happiest moments were because of her and more recently Cari. I wanted her to promise me she would always look out for the boys, my beautiful twin nephews who stole my heart when I first met them when they were just one hour old. I wanted her and her partner to have the best wedding day as they deserved it. I doubted I'd be there to see it though. I truly felt as though my time was coming to an end and the worst thing was no one believed me and there was nothing I could do to convince them otherwise. I could not even pick up my phone to call anyone as I had no strength in my body, I felt like I was dying.

The nurses were back and fore, some lovely, kind, and caring, others seeming indifferent and cold. I dreaded the night when everything seemed so much worse. I prayed my stoma would start working and things would start moving. The bile kept building up in the drainage bag, the smell nauseating and as none of this liquid was being absorbed by my body, I was getting increasingly thirsty and dreamt of glasses of cold lemon squash which were always just out of my reach.

Wednesday 8th March 2017

The next day was just the same, no change, still feeling absolutely dreadful. I was on various drips and was reassured I was doing fine. One nurse even said I needed to make more of an effort! One of the male health assistants, called John, stuck out in my mind. He was big and really friendly so I called him BFJ - Big Friendly John. He always made time for me and provided solace as he chatted to me and assured me this terrible time would end. He explained about the condition ileus and as awful as it was, it would pass. He encouraged me to get out of bed but my blood pressure plummeted and I had to be quickly put back in. I had become quite anaemic and a blood transfusion was arranged. It was to be administered overnight and hopefully this would make me feel better.

The nurse on duty that night was very busy and harassed. Her assistant was a bank nurse who looked clueless, to be honest, which added to the regular nurse's bad mood. I felt afraid. I really didn't think I was going to make it through the night, yet no one seemed to acknowledge how I was feeling. The 'anxious patient' label well and truly tainted anything I had to say – in any event, it was all about numbers and I didn't score enough for any alarms to be triggered. The nurse started to set up the blood for the transfusion and discovered the cannula in my hand had stopped working. This irritated her immensely, as she mumbled, 'This is all I need,' and decided to administer it through the port in my neck. I knew this was being kept in case I needed urgent drugs but when I asked her if she was sure it was ok, she snapped my head off. I apologised and said I was afraid, but she didn't reply and just moved on to the next patient. I could see how busy she was but nonetheless felt so worthless.

In the middle of the night, I called for help. A bank nurse attended, and she spoke little English. I asked her if she could help me. I felt like I was being crushed and asked if she could rub my back or something. She stared blankly at me and handed me the morphine pump. I said I didn't want morphine, I wasn't in acute pain, I just felt I was suffocating as if someone was sitting on my chest. She said nothing, backed out of the room, almost shutting the door, and left. I could not even reach the call bell. I felt I would die that night, alone. Just another poorly patient wheeled off in a body bag in the middle of the night.

Thursday 9th March 2017

I do not remember every detail of this day, the day I nearly died. I do remember noticing the bile in the nasogastric tube was less and this was noted as a positive step. I also remember telling a lovely new health care assistant who had come to help me wash that I felt confused and shivery. She took my temperature which read a worrying 39.8 Celsius which is almost 104 Fahrenheit in old money. She looked concerned and called a nurse who said she would call the doctor. By now, I knew I was deteriorating. I could hear everything but couldn't really speak, I could see but couldn't make sense of it all somehow. A doctor eventually came and mumbled something about antibiotics. Sepsis was mentioned, my heart rate was elevated, my temperature still high, despite paracetamol. I felt so weak I did not want to converse with them or fight my corner. I'd given up, I just wanted to sleep or die, I didn't really care which.

About lunchtime, Andrew arrived, his smiling face hoping to find me better. Shocked when he saw me, he looked so broken as I lay there lifeless. I held his hand with what little strength I had, trying to find the right words that just wouldn't materialise. I was so uncomfortable, I asked him to help me sit up at the edge of the bed. We managed this with some difficulty, and I rested my head on his stomach as he stood in front of me. He put his arms around me and rested his head on top of mine. I could feel his tears run down my back as he told me how much he loved me and how he was going to find the consultant, something wasn't right here.

That moment has always stayed with me as the depth of our love was so apparent. We had had a rocky marriage in some ways. Illness takes many prisoners and had brought many problems and stresses. But here we were, almost knowing our time together was coming to an end and we were clinging on to every second. I knew he could feel what I was thinking. He gently laid me back on the bed whilst he went to look for a nurse. This was such a busy ward and he said there was no one about. He went back out and eventually found someone who said I had been seen by a doctor and they were waiting on antibiotics, the consultant would be around 'at some point', or alternatively, he could ring his secretary and make an appointment.

'I think my wife is dying,' he said but no one listened. He came back in and sat down next to me. He told me he would watch me sleep until the consultant came. I closed my eyes and suddenly it happened - I couldn't breathe. There was no breath left in me and I could not take one to inflate my lungs, I felt as if I had a plastic bag taped over my face.

I gestured to Andrew who hit the panic button and ran out calling for help. The nurse came in and said I was having a panic attack until my SATS suggested something really serious was going on. She called for the crash team and the next thing I recall were lots of people standing and talking all over me. An oxygen mask strapped to my face eased my absolute hunger for air as I heard the words, 'She's minutes from a cardiac arrest.' I could see Andrew being escorted from the room. The rest is a blur of CT scans, a feeling of almost flying down corridors and then being placed in Intensive Care where I was met with doctors and more doctors. Ventilation was mentioned, someone was trying to insert a line in my neck whilst something was forcing air into my lungs.

I vomited profusely, they cut my clothes off and then . . nothing. I had dropped into very welcome unconsciousness.

Chapter 10

The doorbell rang. I could hear someone saying, 'John, John, answer the door, come on, John, answer the door, the bell rang again.' John was not answering the door. I soon realised that John was the person in the bed next to me, why were they telling him to answer the door? I felt confused. Andrew appeared and kissed my forehead, the only bit of my face not obscured by the oxygen mask. He explained it had taken them eight hours to stabilise me, but I was now out of danger. A rather stern consultant came and told me drugs were keeping my kidneys working but as they had removed copious amounts of liquid from my stomach and lungs, I should start to feel better. I couldn't speak, I made gestures with my eyes but I had no idea what had happened here. He said I would stay with them in ICU for a few more days providing I remained OK, and I would then go to CCU – the Critical Care Unit.

I was incredibly thirsty and the desperate need for a cold drink completely consumed me. They gave me a tablespoon of water which was my parched mouth devoured but it almost made things worse. They said as my bodily fluids balanced, the thirst would subside. I couldn't wait, as every molecule of my body was desperate for a drink. I made a plea with God that if only he gave me that cold pint of lemon squash, he could take me as this was a fate worse than death surely. God wasn't listening, though. It seemed no one was listening. As I tried to scream for help, I realised I could not speak, the mask forcing oxygen into my lungs made sure of that. I started to feel myself drifting away, spiralling down and down into an inky black vortex. A desperate voice in my head screamed, 'I don't want to die, I'm not ready to go' but of course no one could hear me. With that, I saw horses, beautiful, colourful carousel horses, dancing around the ceiling. I felt sure they were coming to rescue me. I watched them as they chased each other round and round the edge of the room and with that, I was lifted from the blackness into a different world where I was greeted by a crimson sunset and calming seas, so unbelievably beautiful it brought tears to my eyes. The horses had been sent to save me and take me home. I drifted in and out of consciousness, afraid to let go in case the horses left me behind but for now, they were with me, keeping me safe from the black, coal black, darkness.

As the days passed, my lungs slowly started to improve. The amount of oxygen I needed was reduced and I started to be able to sit up and converse, albeit by writing things down. Andrew was back and fore as was my daughter, her partner, and my sister. I asked about the children and was assured they were all fine. But I blocked them out of my mind as I couldn't bear the sadness of never seeing them again, as I was still convinced I was going to die. It was explained to me I'd aspirated some liquid and my lungs had collapsed. I also had intra-abdominal sepsis, so I was lucky, to have survived at all.

The next day, disaster struck again as one of the drain bags filled with liquid. This meant the repair had failed yet again and I was back to square one. The consultant came to see me, and I could see he was also devastated at this development. He couldn't find the words to reassure me as there just weren't any. I spent the next few days in a state of shock and disbelief. How would I ever come back from this? How many more knocks could I take?

I asked about John and the doorbell. They explained John, in the bed next to me, had been in a coma and they'd been trying to rouse him by saying things that may trigger a memory, like a doorbell or a phone ringing. John had died in the night; he'd never need to worry about the doorbell again. The nurses told me to be positive as despite this setback, where there was life there was hope. I was stabilising and would soon leave ICU.

I was moved into CCU. The nurses were lovely and whilst taking great care of me, asked about my family and life before all of this. I was really struggling mentally and saw a psychologist who said it was normal to feel as I was feeling, having gone through such a trauma and that as my physical health improved, so would my mental health.

That thought plagued me in the dead of night. What if I did not improve physically? What if the fact the repair had failed meant this new fistula would be high output? I couldn't envisage a life on TPN.

I was having daily physio from a young lad named Connor, who arrived to put me through my exercises. He looked so young but had a maturity about him that gave me confidence to start trusting my body again. My task one day was to walk twenty steps to the corridor, with Connor at my side. This seemed like an enormous ask but I had to at least try. The first job was to untangle all the tubes and drips to make sure I didn't trip over which would have been disastrous. I looked into Connor's eyes and he held my hands tightly as he told me to stand and take my first few steps. It felt like walking through glue and I was terrified my lungs were going to pack in again, or something was going to come gushing out of me. The trauma demon was always at work, making me doubt myself every step of the way. But I looked up and thought about the children and getting home and I somehow completed my task, twenty steps there and back. I collapsed into bed as if I had just climbed Everest and thanked Connor for his patience. I told him I may be going back to the colorectal ward, and he said they'd be keeping an eye on me and that, once I could climb a few steps, I'd be homeward-bound. His kindness and optimism made a lasting impression on me, and I felt a sense of accomplishment as I drifted into an exhausted sleep, dreaming of home, family, the cats and doing normal but precious things.

After a week or so in CCU, I had stabilised sufficiently to be returned to the colorectal ward. This frightened me as I had visions of going back into the room where I had nearly met my Maker. I tried in vain to block out these destructive thoughts and concentrated on trying to stand up. The weakness that encompasses you when you have had sepsis and all the other horrors I'd endured, was unimaginable.

Later that day, I was told the return to the ward was imminent and a porter had been requested. The nurses gathered up my belongings and emptied my locker as the wait began. I felt very anxious going back to that environment and the realisation the op to repair the fistula had failed was devastating. When faced with all the recent traumas, the goal posts had moved. When my lungs failed, I just wanted to breathe again unaided; when that happened, I wanted to walk and so on. I couldn't accept staying as I was, but I knew the recovery would be long and protracted, with undoubtedly many hurdles along the way. The trolley arrived and I waved everyone goodbye before the cheery porter started the short journey to the ward.

I arrived at the ward around 6.30pm and was ushered into a side room, thankfully not the room I'd left a few weeks before when my lungs packed in. It was almost handover time, so everyone was rushing about. I was eased into bed and told where the bell was. The nurse left and the automatic light went out, plunging me into darkness. I couldn't find the bell and just sat there and wept, a pity party for one! This was just the last straw!

Sometime later, much to my delight, my favourite healthcare assistant - BFJ – arrived and soon made me feel better. He gave me some sips of water which tasted like pure nectar and told me the nurse would be along soon to give me my 'food'. Not a morsel had past my lips for weeks as I was back on the TPN, the liquid vein feed which was keeping me alive for the second time in as many years. The nurses came and did handover, and I heard the words 'respiratory failure' and 'sepsis' before they checked all the various drips and drains, explaining to the night staff the drain on the left was faecal which reinforced the devastating news that the operation had definitely failed and a new fistula had formed.

I had a fitful night's sleep, thanks to the tick tick tick of the TPN machine. I awoke around 6am to the sound of the water trolley trundling down the corridor. A jug of ice-cold water was plonked on my locker, out of reach which was just as well as I was so thirsty, I would have drunk the whole jug. The daily rituals began and about 11am, the nurse came to change my dressings as one of them was leaking. She took the dressing off the midline scar and I saw my mutilated abdomen in all its glory, the staples desperately trying to keep it all together. Then I noticed it - at the bottom of the scar there was a bulge, it looked like a blood blister. My heart sank as I realised what this could mean.

A doctor attended and prodded it and out spilled a black looking liquid which he said initially was blood. He prodded a bit deeper and the sickeningly familiar sight of brownish bile seeped out and dribbled ominously onto the white sheet of the bed. He told me, quite casually, it looked like another fistula had formed and the rest of my scar may now open up. So not only had the repair op failed, but it had also made things worse! I now had two fistulas with maybe more to follow. How will I ever move on from this? I could feel my brain sort of shutting down, as if refusing to take on any more trauma. I shut my eyes and hoped I'd never wake up.

Chapter 11

I awoke with a start to see my consultant and his entourage standing around my bed. I hate it when that happens, and I try desperately to appear awake and alert but I am still half asleep and in my current state of mind almost disappointed to have awoken to another day of reality. I heard some of the dialogue about how they had attempted to repair the fistula, but I had developed complications again and the repair had failed. I also hear the words 'very anxious' uttered and I felt that somehow, a less anxious person would have just embraced all of this with far more courage than I. He gave instructions to his team about what blood tests to carry out and we finally made eye contact. I knew he was devastated at the outcome. He told me once I was his Everest - I assumed by that he meant the ultimate challenge. But his attempts to fix me had failed and I was losing faith in life in general, but not in him. I knew he was a brilliant surgeon and the nicest consultant and without him I would have probably given up years ago.

I honestly hadn't expected the surgery to go wrong again. I trusted my consultant implicitly and in all my years of surgeries and procedures, I could now see that I had never had really serious complications before. Perhaps I had become complacent, completely underestimating the risks of surgery. At this point however, I had felt there was no choice as the thought of life with a fistula was just not an option for me. I didn't even realise things could go so wrong that you almost die, that some complications cannot be fixed and are so serious you may never eat or drink again. That's one heck of an outcome and had plunged me into a hell I didn't even know was possible, for the second time or was it third? I'd lost count. I never for a minute had I thought surgery could make things worse, but here I was back, not at square one, more like minus 10.

I thought of my old consultant, the one who had repeatedly drained those cysts year after year. There were always doubts as to their origins but of course I never had a definitive answer. In those days, you never challenged your doctor, and when I did ask him, he openly admitted that 'we don't know what it is but we know what it isn't', meaning he knew it wasn't cancer and so everything else was manageable. He used to tell me repeatedly not to have a hysterectomy unless my life was at risk as it would open a 'Pandora's box of problems', undoubtedly replacing one issue with many others. So why did I agree to the hysterectomy? Because I listened to the experts and I'm sure they never expected the outcome to be so bad. But here I was again, having to face up to the fact my life would be plunged into an abyss of uncertainty again.

The weeks passed with the monotony I'd grown accustomed to. As I couldn't eat, I didn't have meals to look forward to so, as everyone else tucked into their lunch, I used to try and go for a walk around the ward, even though I still felt very weak and unwell.

April 23rd was Andrew's birthday and he came to take me to a local park, where I was to meet Annie and Cari. A few hours' leave had been approved and we made the short journey to the park. I remember feeling every bump in the road and part of me just wanted to return to the ward. I didn't feel great but that was nothing new and Andrew had brought a wheelchair for me as even he could see how weak and frail I had become.

We spent a pleasant hour in the park and as Andrew and Annie enjoyed a hot chocolate, I had a sip of water, scared at what hole it would come out from, still so afraid of my own body. They took me back to the ward and I kissed them goodbye, my heart breaking at not being able to go with them. They were off to have a birthday meal in a nearby pub.

A deep sadness filled me as I watched them go, wondering if I would ever eat normally again but more importantly would I ever get the opportunity to really know my beautiful granddaughter. Annie had only ever known me ill, yet until this damned hysterectomy, I truly felt that was behind me and I would have the luxury of growing old disgracefully. But now everything had changed.

I lay on the bed and fell asleep, to be awoken by the trundling of the drugs trolley. I still didn't feel great and was hoping some paracetamol would help. The nurse, however, told me I couldn't have any paracetamol - my liver function tests were dangerously high, and a doctor would come and see me soon. What now? I thought, please, no more problems. I just cannot bear any more. I was still spiking the occasional elevated temperatures and the thought of no paracetamol worried me. I was so sick of being sick.

A young doctor came about 9pm and explained my liver enzymes were extremely high - about five times higher than they should be, so no paracetamol for the foreseeable and I'd have to have a specialised liver scan ASAP. I lay in bed worrying what this meant. If I was somehow intolerant to the TPN (it can have an adverse effect on your liver), it would mean I would literally starve to death. I thought of all the years I'd spent worrying about my 'weight problem' and now I was faced with this unimaginable situation. I closed my eyes and prayed to God to give me strength and help me cope. I hoped he was listening this time.

I made slow progress as weeks merged into months. The MRI on my liver had revealed gallstones and some of the blighters were stuck in my bile duct so this probably was the cause of me feeling unwell and my very abnormal blood test. Things improved slowly as my body started to pick up a bit, the TPN was tweaked to make it gentler on the liver and my body slowly adapted. The nurses decided I needed company and moved me to a four bedder on the other side of the ward. This is always an awkward encounter as everyone waits to greet their new 'cellmate', secretly hoping they are quiet and don't snore. I was introduced to everyone and the lady to my right was called Ann. I immediately took to her as she too had a fistula and I thought it would be good to share experiences.

How wrong I was! Ann did indeed have an abdominal fistula like me. She also had three bags and couldn't eat or drink at all. A few years back, her repair surgery had also gone badly wrong, and she now really struggled with it all. Her husband visited her every day at 2 o'clock on the dot. He was a seemingly quiet man, who walked with a bad limp and a weary expression – however, his face lit up when he saw Ann. They chatted and held hands, sometimes he would hand her half an orange for her to suck on before she would carefully spit out the juices into a receiver, unable to swallow the bitter sweet nectar.

That image haunted me as I realised that could have been me and could well be me in the future. The prospect of never eating or drinking again was a fate worse than death but she seemed to have adapted because, as she said, she had no choice, they were a team and they helped each other through. Other times, I heard her crying behind the curtain as the bags had leaked yet again and she told the nurse for the 100th time, 'I can't do this any longer.'

As I had now been in hospital for seven weeks, Andrew was no longer visiting every day as it was too far and was taking its toll on him mentally and physically, even though he was not working at this time. He had passed any outstanding work onto his electrician colleagues, leaving him free to concentrate on our situation. We agreed communicate via our iPads, and he would just visit at weekends. It was hard but his visits had become quite stressful for both of us as he always hoped for improvement in my condition but was usually disappointed as I had reached a point of stability but nothing more. He grasped at every snippet of positivity whereas I almost couldn't bear to be hopeful for fear of being let down again. It felt like we were just growing further and further apart, yet somehow, at the same time, clinging on to each other with every fibre

73

in our bodies. In the last few months, we had cried, laughed, cried some more, prayed, begged but not given up. We would fight on for each other and our loved ones. This thing called a fistula that had come into my life and wreaked total carnage, we would not let this win. It, of course, had other ideas.

Day fifty and I awoke to find the fistula bag half full of bright red blood. My heart sank to my proverbial boots as I dreaded having to deal with more bad news. I showed the nurse who didn't seem fazed and told me to tell the doctors as they were on their way round. The team arrived and pleasantries over, I showed them the bloody liquid in the fistula bag. The doctor said blood wasn't always a bad thing and they would keep an eye. 'Always keeping an eye' of course was a good thing, as they didn't seem that concerned but it also meant more anxiety and more trauma for me as the fear of what this thing would do next was heightened. Why can't it just heal? Why didn't I know that not all wounds heal, even when you are otherwise healthy? I just do not understand this.

By day sixty, things had settled and they wanted to try me on food, which terrified me. The nurses said, with their usual nonchalant attitude, that there is only one way to find out how bad the fistula is and that is to eat food They say it with such a 'matter of fact' attitude that it feels harsh and cuts through me like a knife. To them, it's nothing but to me it's everything. I knew enough about this situation to realise if I can't eat enough calories to sustain me, I will have to go home on parenteral nutrition (PN). The alternative was I'd slowly but surely starve to death. Andrew and I have always shared a love of decent food and wine and to be denied that would be hard enough but to not be able to drink or eat at all would be, and is, just torture. So they said I had to start eating small amounts and if I became ill, then I would be put back on the PN. Words are so easy when it's not happening to you. The feed enters your body through a vein by your heart. That in itself is fraught with danger but keeps people alive. I wondered sometimes if that's alive but not actually living. I talked to Annie online about it all and she said she would rather have me on PN than not at all. Even if I never left the house again, me just being there was enough - reading books to Cari and being Aunty to the boys - that was enough. I was enough and she needed me to be there. That filled my heart with love and I desperately tried to bury all the negative thoughts and fears, knowing that I had to somehow find the strength to deal with all of this.

I started on cups of tea which progressed to crackers and cheese. It was like eating cardboard as I didn't feel hungry and had no appetite because I was still on PN. Of the two, it was drinking I missed the most and having experienced extreme thirst on this journey, a drink was never far away from me.

As the days became weeks, I became more confident on the food front. Of course, what goes in must come out and the constant measuring of the output from the fistula tube was stressful and pretty frightening as I knew if it increased, it was bad news, but so far so good. I worried about what was going on inside. Was it still leaking slowly, just waiting to build up and cause sepsis as the toxins escape into my body? I wished I could switch my mind off, but the anxiety and trauma were never far away, especially being in this environment for so long. I'd seen too much, heard too much and now I feared what the future held. The surgery that was supposed to set me free has imprisoned me again, only this time it's harder as yet another massive knock has dented my already depleted confidence. Ignorance is definitely bliss sometimes.

The days passed and I thought things were going ok until I woke up yet again to a lot of blood in the fistula bag. On further examination, a deep hole had reopened. As usual, I was devastated. We saw the consultant and he said it was ok, at least he didn't say 'it's fine'! I again expressed my absolute disappointment at what was happening and that I still couldn't get my head around it all. He told me I'm thinking too far ahead and in three months, everything could look different. He wanted me to go home if I wanted to, but I just wasn't sure I was well enough. But again, most people leave hospital when they are still unwell as it's a known fact you recover better at home. But I still had this demon within me, it was like a cancer burrowing away at me, so I couldn't see how I would recover as it was just going to get worse until it was completely settled, if it ever did settle. I thought of my fistula friend Ann who, on the outside, was positive and grateful, yet told me it was a living hell on the inside. I wasn't sure I could stand it here much longer though, as it was soul destroying to see and hear all these horror stories.

I had a visit from the chaplain. She was quirky-looking with long pigtails and a sunny smile, probably in her sixties. We had a long chat about everything and nothing. She had such a soft voice I could barely hear her. I told her I felt lost and broken by the events of the last two years and she understood having 'been hit in the face by a plank' a few times herself. She said this will pass and I must look after me now, with rest, meditation, good nutrition, and gentle exercise. I did that before though, and nothing changed, I never healed. She held my hand and reminded me how loved I am and how I will learn to accept and cope. It's like a grief, she said, because I have lost my health and must come to terms with that. It may not be forever. Some people she sees have no hope, but I did and I had to cling onto that for my lovely family and friends. I knew all of this but still felt overwhelmed by sadness and regret.

I also had a visit from one of the Outreach team – that's the team that saved me on 9th March when my lungs failed. I told him I wasn't sure what had happened and so he explained. This was the first time someone medical had actually explained what had happened to me. Up to now, questions went unanswered or evaded, probably because my mental state was so fragile. His honesty at how close I had come to dying was very sobering and, for a short while at least, made me feel gratitude and not absolute horror at my situation.

He explained that the weekend of surgery had left me physically exceptionally low and therefore vulnerable. In addition, my bowel had stopped working and I developed ileus when my intestines stopped working so everything was on stop. My liver, however, had continued to produce copious amounts of bile which now had nowhere to go and so they had been aspirating it off my stomach all week via the horrible nasal tube. On the day of the respiratory failure, the amount aspirated had reduced massively but unbeknown to anyone, the bile was collecting in my stomach, to the point I aspirated some into my lungs, causing them to collapse. He told me how they had pumped out two litres in Intensive Care which saved my life but by then, my kidneys had started to fail, requiring more intervention from the highly skilled staff. I was lost for words and thanked him for everything. My words somehow just didn't seem enough. He wished me well and off he went. I've never forgotten him.

Day seventy - I developed a fever in the night and the doctor on call put a cannula in my hand, ready for antibiotics whilst waiting on blood tests. If I needed antibiotics, I would not be going home as they needed to be intravenously administered for at least five days. I was feeling OK that morning but that familiar shivery feeling was there in the background. My consultant said he wanted me out of this environment, as it was time to go home. I wanted to go home to sleep better and walk a bit, eat better and feel happier. I wanted to take the pressure off Andrew who had to drive to see me and continue to run the ship back home whilst, he said, his heart was breaking. I wanted to see my loved ones. It was the twins' eighth birthday on the Wednesday. They would have been so disappointed if I didn't make it, I've always been there for them since the day they were born. Plus my beautiful Cari who came into my life at the darkest of times but made the sun shine again.

Plus, of course, my poor mother must have been wondering what had happened to me. Even though she had no idea who I was most of time, she knew I was someone kind whom she could trust. Her face would light up when she had visitors and she'd tell her fellow residents I was her sister or mother, even. It didn't matter to me though, as it gave her some happiness, albeit short lived. I wish I could have made her understand the reality of our torrid situation. I hoped she didn't think I'd abandoned her.

Last but not least, I wanted to see my forever friends, some of whom I had known for over thirty years and had been with me every step of the way, always there with a kind listening ear or a late-night message of support and encouragement. But as much I wanted to go home, I was terrified of what might happen as I just did not trust my own body anymore. In fact, I didn't trust anything much which made for a very difficult life

Chapter 12

Monday 8th May 2017

I was expecting to be in hospital a few more days at least because of the recent fever but the blood tests had not indicated an active infection so no more antibiotics for now. I felt reasonable and the Sister seemed to be on a mission to discharge people and I was on her hit list. I said how worried I was about going home and she said they weren't babysitters - she certainly had a way with words! I wanted to explain how my GP practice had been taken over by the health board and was run by locums, none of whom had any experience of this type of fistula. My last visit, before this latest surgical disaster, had resulted in the young female GP insisting, rather aggressively, she examine my back passage as that's 'the only place you could have a fistula'. I tried to explain mine was in my abdomen, but she looked at me as if I was insane. I left in tears and vowed never to return. I didn't bother explaining all of this to the Ward Sister as it would have made no difference. It was time to leave.

The registrar came round, accompanied by the said Sister, and we discussed how I was doing. My blood tests were ok, the fistula was doing what they do, there was no real reason to keep me in hospital. He seemed a little reluctant to let me go but Sister was having none of it. It was decided the central line would be removed asap and I could go home later in the afternoon.

They arrived shortly after with their kit to remove the line. I've had this done before and it's not the best experience, but any messing with your jugular vein isn't exactly ever going to be fun. The Registrar (6'6" in both directions, one very scary-looking man with yellowing eyes and wearing a leather coat that was way too small for him) administered lots of local anaesthetic which stung like mad. After what seemed like a nano second, he proceeded to stick needles in me to check if I could feel the sharpness. I could. He waited a little longer and I said it still felt mildly sharp but he seemed to be getting impatient, so I didn't want to upset him, as he literally had my life in his very large podgy hands. He started cutting and I could feel and then see the warm blood running down my side onto the crisp white sheet beneath me. My curling toes alerted them to the fact I was very tense, and they suggested gas and air would probably help. I was soon deeply inhaling the laughing gas which did have a calming effect and made the pushing, prodding and then stitching slightly more bearable. Once the procedure was over, I had to lie still for an hour whilst they periodically checked for excessive bleeding. Anxiety kicked in as I hoped he hadn't made any mistakes and accidentally severed my jugular, always a drama but I now knew how easy it was to die.

I left the ward at 4pm. My wheelchair was piled high with all the trappings of the previous three months, and I turned to say my goodbyes but there was no one there. I often felt some of the staff resented my presence; after all, I wasn't from the area and they felt I could be treated closer to home. But I wasn't going to ponder on that now, I was homeward bound at last.

We made the long journey home in relative silence. Andrew reached out for my hand at every opportunity, silently telling me, 'It will be ok.' Every time a sad song came on the radio, he turned it off as he knew it would make me cry. Deep down inside, I didn't think it would ever be ok again. I knew I was nowhere near better and in fact there was every likelihood things would actually get worse for me.

But now, though, I was also becoming acquainted with the world of 'toxic positivity' - where negativity wasn't an option and I had to be upbeat all the time and thankful for the constant false reassurances rather than the sometimes harsh reality that proper empathy provided. My husband, for one, had never been comfortable with negative emotions and was something of an ostrich where problems were concerned. I had always done the worrying in this relationship. His intentions were good, of course, but left me with a feeling of alienation and disconnection as I forced a smile, knowing deep down he had absolutely no concept of how I was feeling, or if he did, he had the ability to lock those feelings away in the back of his mind. It was more manageable for him if I buried my true emotions way below the surface like a simmering volcano because it made him feel better. So that is what I did, the mask well and truly painted on as I tried to get on with my 'new normal'. I wasn't allowed to talk about the fistula, he would put his hands over his ears to block it all out, he just could not handle it. Maybe the old normal wasn't that great after all, perhaps I should be open to new possibilities with this big life change. My mind pondered on this thought but I needed stability now and everything in my life suddenly felt anything but.

A few days after I got home, as I was lying on the bed, having just come out of the shower, I decided to have a proper look at my wounded abdomen. Up to now, Andrew had had the honour of changing the bags, as I just couldn't bear to look. He was very good at it, in fairness but I couldn't bear to see the sadness in his face, so the whole process was carried out with my eyes shut.

The phone rang and ironically it was my consultant which really surprised me. He knew I was very worried about leaving hospital and had said he was going to ring but I never expected him to, he was exceptionally busy.

On hearing his voice, I broke down and all the sadness and fear came flooding out. I was just about able to tell him through my uncontrollable blubber how devastated I was, how it all looked worse than before and how I was having flashbacks of the respiratory failure and kept thinking it was going to happen again. He made the usual noises about 'early days' and 'doing fine' but his words somehow sounded hollow. He didn't have to live this and the more I was learning about this 'catastrophic outcome' to surgery, the more it was becoming apparent that this may be me for life.

I needed to know why this had happened, not once or twice but three times. Three times the surgery had caused my bowel to fall apart. Healthy tissues do not disintegrate, even if they are accidentally pierced, they often heal. I remember many a time during long hospital stays hearing doctors tell patients, usually elderly, they had a little perforation but it would heal. Why wasn't mine healing?

I looked up the reasons for why this could happen – radiation damage, Crohn's disease, diverticular disease, to name a few, but I didn't tick any of those boxes. Yes, I'd had Crohn's disease (but I was even doubting that now) but my consultant had said repeatedly this was not driven by Crohn's, it was just bad luck. I just couldn't accept that. Surgery surely wasn't about luck, it was about the amazing skills of these doctors, yet with me things had gone badly wrong again - there must be an underlying cause, yet no one could or would answer my questions.

He agreed, during the phone call, that once I was stronger, he would arrange for me to see a colleague of his in London. He was also pleased I was waiting for mental health support, albeit on a very long waiting list. In the meantime, 'The Sword of Damocles' would continue hanging over me. A fistula has no set pattern and is very unpredictable. It directs the bowel contents to a safe place, thereby keeping me alive, but if it stops working and the bowel contents leak inside, I will become very sick very quickly so, as much as I hate it, at the moment I need it just to survive.

Andrew couldn't wait to return to work. By his own admission, he really struggled as my carer and needed interaction with people outside the home. He started a new job with a construction company so now worked full time, coming home exhausted. It also meant that, from 9am, a constant stream of parcels containing electrical components arrived at our door, which was difficult if I was mid bag change or catching up on much-needed sleep. It felt like he preferred to be in work than be with me. In some ways, this was understandable; hardly the retirement we had hoped for, after a lifetime of my surgeries. The hysterectomy was to be my panacea whereas in fact it had become my apocalypse. He wanted his wife back, not the person left by this mutilating surgery. He never said as much but he didn't have to, his silent sadness spoke volumes.

In his defence, he has dealt with this for all our married life and he has been amazing in so many ways. I remember when I was twenty-six and the bowel disease really took hold, he had to practically carry me to bed every night as I became more and more poorly. But all that stopped when I had my stoma, it restored our lives, but this surgery had destroyed it. He now returned home from work every day, hoping for a miracle that I'd somehow be getting better, and life would be back to normal. It just wasn't happening and I found dealing with his disappointment almost worse than dealing with my own. The void between us was growing. He just didn't seem capable of handling this and I was sinking deeper and deeper into depression, fuelled by fear of my own body and its seemingly constant desire to kill me.

In September 2017, we made the journey to London to see an expert colleague of my consultant. We decided to travel by train as we hoped it would be less stressful for both of us. We had planned our trip and hoped to go up The Shard for afternoon tea.

We started the journey from Paddington Station to our hotel by Underground but it soon became apparent I was not up to it so we resorted to a taxi. We arrived at the Harley Street clinic feeling quite nervous but grateful for the opportunity to see this expert in all things bowel. He was a lovely man and instantly put us at ease. Having read my notes, he was surprised I looked so well and had expected me to be in a wheelchair, which worried me somewhat. I asked him some tough questions about life and life expectancy with a fistula and he said ideally it would be fixed at some point. He told me he had one patient, now elderly, who did live with it but I would obviously be better off without it. He could offer no real reassurance about life expectancy and agreed it could make me ill very quickly but then again it could all settle down and become nothing more than a nuisance. He offered to come to Wales to assist my surgeon when the time for repair came but stressed it would be at least two years hence, to give everything time to settle again. We left the clinic about 6pm on the autumn afternoon, the weather was perfect – dry and sunny. I had wanted to go down Oxford Street but just didn't have the energy so we returned to the hotel. Our planned meal out was also cancelled as I just felt too exhausted. We ordered pizza in the room and spent the evening relaxing and talking about the appointment.

We awoke next morning to the sound of sirens; I knew we were in central London, but this seemed excessive as fleets of emergency vehicles flew past our hotel. We went down for breakfast and caught sight of the news - 'London comes to standstill following terrorist attack.' We soon learned that a terrorist bomb had indeed gone off in Parsons Green on the District Line, the very same line we had been on yesterday. Chaos reigned as the Underground was essentially shut down while information was gathered. Our planned visit to The Shard was obviously cancelled and we even wondered if we would be able to get home.

We eventually managed to get a taxi and paid an exorbitant amount to get to Paddington, owing to all the delays and diversions. But we eventually made it and were glad to be out of all the chaos and on our way home to our little bungalow which was fast becoming my sanctuary and the only place I felt safe.

A few weeks after seeing the London expert, it was my fifty-seventh birthday. Historically on birthdays and all family events, I was the host, and this was no exception. Family were arriving at six pm so I would have all day to sort everything out. One thing I had learned was how I now had to pace myself as once my batteries deplete, sitting down and having a cuppa just doesn't recharge them. A few friends told me about the spoon theory which is a popular metaphor used in disability circles. The theory uses spoons as a visual way to explain how much energy someone has throughout the day - the more you do, the less spoons you have until they are all used up.

Let's say you have twelve spoons. In an average day, you might want to wake up, brush your teeth, wash your face, get dressed, eat breakfast, go to the doctors, come home, make and eat dinner, change into your pyjamas. Some of these tasks, like brushing your teeth, may only use up one spoon, while going to the doctors could use up six spoons. This leaves you with no, or few, spoons for everything else and there's no way you can make a few spoons stretch that far. Once you run out of spoons, you have no choice but to rest, or otherwise push through 'borrowing' spoons from the following day, which of course means you start the next day already missing some spoons.

My spoons run out very quickly and there is no coming back until the next day, or maybe the day after. So, by the time everyone arrived, I was tired but happy to celebrate my birthday with the people I love. We had a finger buffet prepared by Andrew and the Prosecco was flowing. The children played happily and watched as I opened my presents. Everyone went to such an effort and my main present was a lovely pink iPad which everyone had contributed to. I was delighted, and even more so when it was all set up and ready to go. Andrew made a joke about 'how my head would now be permanently stuck in that thing' and I agreed with him, secretly thinking how it would give me a new focus and I could finally start writing my book! Everyone left about nine and after clearing up, I collapsed into bed, not even needing my meditation app to get me to sleep, all my spoons well and truly spent. It had been a good day, a day when I felt so grateful that I was still around.

Chapter 13

After ten months, I had my first appointment with a consultant psychiatrist. I'd been through months of assessments, and I don't think they really knew what to do with me. They thought it was Post Traumatic Stress Disorder (PTSD) but then again, the trauma wasn't over, so they were unsure whether to try Cognitive Behavioural Therapy which helps you manage your problems by changing the way you think or behave, or some other therapy. In the end, I was sent to the top - a consultant psychiatrist who specialised in many areas of mental health. She was to assess me to see what, in her opinion, my diagnosis was. Once that was established, a plan of treatment would commence. She explained therapy didn't always work in cases where the trauma had been so great, and it may not achieve the desired outcome but she would do her best to help me. I felt an instant connection with her, she understood what I was saying and didn't marginalise my thoughts and feelings. I felt heard and worthy of her time, which in turn gave me the strength and the confidence to open up to her. At last, someone was listening.

The first few appointments were really about my childhood and early life, and I was pleased to report no demons there. I'd had a perfectly happy childhood filled with love and was an only child until I was nearly thirteen, when my mother had a baby. Despite that being a bit of a shock, I was so happy to finally have a sister. Life did change somewhat then as I had started in grammar school, so it was a bit odd to have a baby sister. I was frequently mistaken for her mother as, at 13 years old, I was very tall for my age. This had affected my confidence as I towered over my peers and spent my weekends pushing my baby sister around as both my parents worked, but I was happy enough and cannot remember anything negative from that time.

I told her I felt my anxiety started when I developed Crohn's disease when I was twenty-six. Annie was just two and Andrew in the Royal Navy. It had been difficult managing alone with a serious illness, a full-time job and a husband who was away a lot. I'd relied heavily on my parents for support but by then, my father had developed emphysema and my maternal grandmother was seriously ill. It was only many years later that I realised how my mother endured the most of everyone's problems. How I wished I'd been more openly appreciative of her. She was not one to show affection and often seemed quite irritable. It is only now as an adult that I can truly appreciate why, juggling way too many plates with very little help or acknowledgment.

I also explained to the therapist how I had had surgery every year of the last thirty years of my life, as first Crohn's and then endometriosis took hold and continued to wreak havoc in my pelvis. It had understandably imposed restrictions on our lives and in some ways Andrew and I had drifted apart whilst trying to carve out a life so controlled by my illness. He had his job and his hobbies including a huge love of rugby and the socialising that went with it. I also worked full time and had my own circle of friends. It was becoming apparent we were hugely different beings with different needs and dreams.

My daughter, however, grew up to be the best daughter we could have asked for. She was the kindest, most empathetic child and had an absolute love of animals. We had several pets, and our home was never without a cat or two, her favourite probably being Pusscat who lived to a ripe old age of twenty-one and was Annie's shadow. Even though her childhood was undoubtedly affected by my ill health, I hope and pray she always felt loved. It was a very proud day for us when she received her PhD in Computer Science and we had the honour of calling her Dr!

The therapist asked me to talk about that good memory and I explained how we'd had a lovely celebration in a nearby hotel. All Annie's close family were there, as were the twins who were barely toddling. I'd had my fair share of champagne and felt relaxed and happy. She received several gifts and I remember we gave her a carved love spoon which she adored.

Of course, this was before the surgical trauma when, despite having a stoma, I used to love dressing up and going out. I explained how my relationship with Annie was strong and watching her develop as a wonderful mother was one of the greatest joys in my life. I hoped that despite my shocking health, I had got something right.

The therapist soon noticed my worryingly low self-esteem and she wanted to 'explore that'. She said she saw me as a courageous person who should be proud of all my achievements, despite the fact my health had been a constant battle. But I didn't see it like that and felt quite awkward and embarrassed at her words.

The sessions were arduous and difficult but I was learning a lot about myself and some of the decisions, both good and bad, I had made in life. When it came to talking about the surgery going so wrong, Andrew joined the sessions. She felt it would help us communicate as a couple without him being able to put the shutters up and pretend it hadn't happened or walk off in a temper. I told her the surgery going wrong was without doubt the biggest disappointment of our life. My gut feeling had always been not to have the surgery but I was in a cleft stick, and I did what I thought was right at the time. But the consequences had been life-changing. It wasn't just the damaging physical outcome of those adverse surgical events – what was equally damaging was that no one acknowledged the seriousness of what had occurred and being told constantly to be grateful I was still alive. Of course I was grateful but I was also extremely sad at what I had lost but that reaction, it seemed to me, just wasn't allowed.

To make matters worse, Andrew believed the consultant and not me, so if he said I was doing fine, then that was it. It didn't matter how I felt or what was happening. As far as he was concerned, I was fine and I needed to just get on with things and stop complaining about the horrific symptoms I was dealing with daily. He often used to say how people had it far worse than me, as if I didn't know that, but it didn't make my problems any the less important.

It took me years to realise that, when the consultant said, 'You're doing fine,' he should have added, 'for a fistula patient.' Compared to other people with an enterocutaneous fistula, I probably was 'doing fine' but compared to a 58-year-old previously reasonably healthy, fully functioning normal woman, I most certainly was not.

My husband, being a typical male, told the therapist how he wanted to fix me but as this problem couldn't be fixed, he just wanted me to accept, move on and not talk about it. He did not see the point as talking would change nothing. He wanted us to make the best of what we had. As I was able to tell him in the safe space the therapy environment offered, how could I when I felt mutilated as a woman and broken as a person? Plus, everything we had previously enjoyed doing as a couple had been cruelly taken away. I had to now live a different life with the same husband, one who really struggled with the husbandly cocktail of love, duty and absolute mind-numbing boredom that life as a carer demanded. He needed a lot more than his now-disabled wife could give him. He felt therapy was making things worse for us and wanted to stop going. Something else we disagreed on.

The therapist told us early on in our sessions that what had happened to me was life-changing. To have such serious, permanent complications that threatened the most basic functions of eating and drinking, from a surgery that essentially may not have even been needed, was in her words 'crazy making' and we must be prepared for life to never be as it was. It may be that we would be spending the rest of our lives apart, as many couples just weren't able to deal with the trauma. I just wanted him to drop anchor and say, 'I'm here for you and I will help you through, no matter what that takes.' But he just couldn't deal with the prospect of me never getting better and was almost more determined than ever not to allow my illness to affect his life any more than it had to. Maybe it was me who was selfish for expecting more from him but at this point, I didn't know what to believe or think anymore.

Even though I was only supposed to see the therapist for six weeks, the appointments continued for several years. I was diagnosed with PTSD and severe anxiety and even though talking about it helped me, I didn't seem to recover, probably because the demon fistula was still there and making his presence known every day. The therapist felt I needed answers to enable me to move on but there were no answers, it was just one of those things. I found that hard to accept and I knew deep down I would find it difficult to just stop looking.

I revisited the forum dealing with my type of fistula (Enterocutaneous), always hopeful for positive stories of hope and acceptance or some medical breakthrough that would bring our nightmare to an end. It still only had a handful of members and they all seemed in a far worse state than I was. Many of them unable to eat and drink and fed permanently by parenteral nutrition, often hooked up to two bags 24/7, one to feed them and one to take away all their waste. It was surely a completely miserable existence but most of them, unlike me, had had serious illness or cancers that had caused the fistula, so they remained grateful to be alive and had found ways to adapt and get some pleasure from life. That gave me hope. I also decided to re-join the other forum which had thousands of members, most of whom had different types to me but not exclusively. I became friendly with a few of the members and even met one of the ladies in a local coffee shop as she lived fairly near me.

We decided to share stories in the hope it would be cathartic for both of us. Susie explained her problems started after the difficult birth of her first child. A hastily performed forceps delivery resulted in a large episiotomy which was both extremely painful and traumatic. Shortly after her son was born and all the post-delivery pain and bruising had settled, she noticed she was having problems emptying her bowels and these problems continued for many years. Indeed, it was only when her second child was born, some three years later, that she was referred to various specialities until finally a rectocele was discovered. (A rectocele is a weakness that develops in the wall separating the vagina and rectum, most often after pregnancy and childbirth especially where deliveries had required an episiotomy). She underwent several surgeries to try and repair the rectocele and as a result of the final surgery, sixteen years after the birth of her son, she developed a fistula.

She had surgery to place a stitch called a seton which is supposed to act as a drain. It works well for some but in Susie's case, it did not prevent infections and caused extreme pain, requiring antibiotics repeatedly.

After three years and several failed repair procedures, she went to St Mark's Hospital in London which is a centre of excellence for bowel problems. She was advised to have a colostomy in an attempt to rest the lower bowel and heal the fistula. With much trepidation, she agreed to go ahead and had her surgery in 2019. She found life with a stoma challenging, what with the frequent bag leaks and the inevitable spontaneous noises over which there is no control, but she soldiered on, hopeful that this would finally leave her fistula free!

The fistula did eventually heal and she was able to have her stoma reversed at the start of this year.

The whole experience has left her with ongoing physical and emotional issues. She explained she feels like she is on some kind of emotional rollercoaster, experiencing flashbacks from the various surgeries to some of the very uncaring 'care' she received. As she is still in pain, it is impossible to just forget it happened. It's been an awful experience which she has shared with many of her friends. I agreed wholeheartedly with Susie when she found most people could not conceptualise what it's like to live with constant pain, uncertainty and downright misery that life with a fistula can bring.

Susie is now fifty, a mum of two, wife, friend, school governor and clinical psychologist and currently works in a cancer centre.

We both found the conversation emotional and many a tear was shed. Before we parted, she showed me the tattoo she'd had done, just after the colostomy operation. It showed a lady dancing in the rain and her inspiration for it came from the saying, 'Life is not just about waiting for the storm to pass, it's about learning to dance in the rain'. The tattoo is a permanent reminder of her ability to cope with adversity.

I also spoke to Rebecca, another active forum member and moderator. Rebecca explained she had always had problems with her bottom! From haemorrhoids to fissures to constipation, there was always something going on down there that shouldn't be. Finally in 2013, she was diagnosed with an anal fistula, something she'd never heard of. It was repaired fairly easily without too much disruption to life, and she thought that was the end of the story. However, a few years later, and just six weeks before her wedding, she developed awful pain in her left buttock which the GP said was an abscess that required surgery. With the wedding imminent, she refused the surgery and opted to keep things at bay by taking antibiotics. By the time the wedding was over, she was in agony and the surgery then proved to be very invasive, leaving her with a large open wound that required daily packing. Hardly the start of married life she had dreamt of! Things got worse when the wound didn't heal and an MRI now indicated a much more complex fistula. She was further devastated to be given the diagnosis of Crohn's disease, a lifelong chronic illness for which she would require strong medication and possibly frequent surgeries. She tried to hide her problems from friends as she found it too embarrassing to talk about them, often saying she had a bad back whereas, inside, she was really struggling with it all and in so much pain she could barely sit down. Thankfully, she too discovered the 'Abscess/fistula support for women' group and the relief was enormous. A safe platform where she could share her story with women going through the same ordeal was just what she needed. Finally, she told me, the sadness, despair and loneliness started to fade which eventually led her to a place where acceptance could begin. Rebecca and a few other members of the support group started a 'Fistula Awareness' group. They have created patient information leaflets and videos with the aim to help patients and their carers/employers. It's fully endorsed by a top UK colorectal surgeon and provides much needed support to other sufferers. She explained she will probably have problems for the rest of her life, but she's accepted that, and she feels it's made her a better and far more empathetic person.

Their stories were so humbling and even though my fistula is physiologically different, there were many similarities. Both have a significant impact on daily life and a massive challenge both physically and emotionally. The Cinderella of health conditions for which there is so little awareness or support, yet the effect on people's lives is just enormous.

Chapter 14

May 2017

There was some nice weather forecast. I could see Andrew was becoming really depressed, and who could blame him? My health was as stable as it was ever going to be, so I suggested we try a little holiday. He nearly fell of his chair in shock that I should suggest such a thing as he knew I struggled leaving the house, let alone going on holiday. I could see, however, by his suddenly sparkly eyes that he loved the idea and was soon researching and booking before I changed my mind!

A few days later, (having changed my mind several times, in my head at least), we set off. We had booked a small cottage overlooking the Cader Idris Mountain range, in southern Snowdonia, near the town of Dolgellau in North Wales.

I was understandably nervous and checked several times where the nearest hospitals were and of course they were miles away. I knew I had to step back into life before it was too late, yet I had to dig very deep into my courage pot not to cancel and stay within the confines of my little bungalow where I felt safe and secure.

The journey took about four hours, and the radio provided a very welcome distraction from the anxiety demon in my head. As we approached our destination, the scenery was spectacular, the only company on the winding roads a few sheep and an occasional car. A frequent 'tap tap tap' on my abdomen told me my bags were fine, all was good. We arrived at the cottage and went inside. It was certainly cosy but also very welcoming and homely. There was a balcony with a table and chairs, simply perfect for sharing a bottle of wine. Maybe, just maybe, I would have a glass.

Andrew decided to go off exploring within minutes of arriving so, after preparing his evening meal, I went to sit on the balcony. The afternoon sun bathed our little home from home in its warm light and I shut my eyes and embraced the heat on my skin. I felt peaceful and at ease and enjoyed a little doze or a 'nanna nap', as Andrew would joke whenever I nodded off in the middle of the day, which seemed to be a frequent occurrence of late.

Sometime later, I was awoken by the sound of the door slamming and realised he was back - think bull in a china shop - they don't call him Bumpy for nothing! He came to see where I was and to my surprise, made us a lovely cup of tea. He'd bought some scones from a nearby shop which we ate hungrily, having not eaten since breakfast. Later that evening, after we had some food, we sat and watched the sun set and yes, I did have a glass of ice-cold Prosecco. We held hands and as we looked out at the view, I knew we had made the right decision. A life was possible with a fistula after all, and I was determined to enjoy every minute of this time away.

The next morning, another surprise awaited me. He had booked us on the Snowdonia Railway, and we were going to the top! For me, this would be quite an achievement, totally out of my comfort zone and I once again fought hard to keep the anxiety demon at bay. We made our way to Llanberis Station. As the weather was really hot, we sat and enjoyed an ice cream and watched all the families waiting for the train to arrive. We boarded around 11am onto a cramped and boiling hot carriage! But as soon as we started our journey, the welcome cooling breeze drifted through, and I relaxed a little. 'Tap tap tap' told me all was ok but here I was, about to make a journey to the top of Snowdon with just a few emergency supplies in my handbag. I looked out of the window and took in the amazing views. It felt like a different world to what I had become accustomed to.

We reached the top and went to the café for a much-needed cold drink. To go to the very top of Snowdon meant a further walk up some rather precarious steps so I decided to stay put whilst Andrew went ahead. I sat outside and took in the amazing scenery, so happy I'd taken the plunge.

A man came and sat next to me and his very friendly demeanour unnerved me a little. He was about my age and explained a trip up Snowdon was on his bucket list and he was so glad he'd made the effort. We were soon chatting like old friends. His name was Dennis and he was a very interesting man. As he left, he took hold of my hand and said, 'Look for the beauty in everything, it will make your journey easier.' And off he went.

I felt a chill rush through me as I hadn't really told him about my nightmare, yet his words resonated so deeply with me. Since all this happened, I'd been so traumatised that all I could see were the bad things in life which had left me pretty dead between the eyes. This had to be a turning point for us. I could see Andrew calling me from the coffee shop and I went to join him. I told him about my encounter with Insightful Dennis and he said he didn't see me talking to anyone or he'd have come to join us. He loved a chat and would have liked Dennis. I looked around to see if I could find him to introduce Andrew to him, but he was nowhere to be seen and was not on the return train which was rather odd.

The journey down seemed quicker, and I could tell Andrew was now getting bored and hungry. Sometimes he was like a 10-year-old boy, constantly needing excitement. He wanted to go out for a meal, whereas I didn't but agreed as it was, after all, his holiday too. Food was still a massive problem for me and at home, we ate different things and often in separate rooms which wasn't good for any relationship. I saw food as a threat just as I had done in hospital. I had soon learnt that food stimulated the fistula and the more that came out of the fistula, the longer I'd have to stay in hospital. That fear had never really left me as the output was, in many ways, the indicator of how bad things were inside.

Nevertheless, I had to eat and so we found a restaurant nearby and ordered our meals. Andrew chose a ribeye steak and I asked if I could have a starter as my main. The waitress looked a bit confused but agreed and so I ordered a prawn cocktail. We couldn't order wine as I wasn't driving at this point, so we had a jug of iced water, much to Andrew's chagrin.

The meals arrived and the portions were just huge. I had the most enormous plate of prawns you'd ever seen. She'd obviously misunderstood my request and presented me with a main size portion of prawn cocktail. Just seeing that amount of food set my heart racing, but we got through it, although I only managed a few mouthfuls with Andrew polishing off the rest. To make up for it, I ordered a cappuccino and some strawberry cheesecake which was delicious and made up for the Prawn Horror Plate. I was glad to get back to our cosy cottage and relax. We had some wine on the balcony and went to bed. I could feel my abdomen gurgling and making all sorts of weird noises but I put my meditation app on and drifted off into a deep sleep, remembering Insightful Dennis's words – look for the beauty in everything, it will make your journey easier . . .

We started the journey home the next day and were both relieved our short holiday had been a success. Relieved because the last few years had really taken its toll on us, but this proved we could still have a life despite the fistula. The sun was still shining as we arrived home. We parked in the drive and composed ourselves before beginning the task of emptying the car and unpacking. Andrew hated this job and I wondered how long it would be before the inevitable bickering would begin again!

Chapter 15

In March 2018, I awoke with a severe pain in my eye, deep in my eye socket, like the worst headache ever, but localised over one eye. What now? I thought and started on yet another rollercoaster looking for answers that didn't seemingly exist.

The GP told me to go to the optician who immediately referred me to the hospital. I was diagnosed with either aggressive episcleritis, a painful inflammatory eye condition, or even the more serious condition scleritis which was sight-threatening. My only experience of eye problems was the odd bout of conjunctivitis. I had never even heard of this condition. The hospital doctors told me that it was a manifestation of my Crohn's disease. I tried to explain that I didn't have active Crohn's and this was a very recent development but it all fell on deaf ears. As far as they were concerned, it was definitely Crohn's-related and they would write to my gastroenterologist. I tried to explain I didn't have a gastroenterologist as I hadn't had active Crohn's for thirty-five years. They said, in an almost patronising way, 'So you had Crohn's, then you had a fistula which is also a manifestation of Crohn's and now you have an inflammatory eye condition which again is a complication of Crohn's, yet you think it's not Crohn's?' I tried to explain it wasn't just me that thought that but my consultant, but no one was interested. This conversation was to be repeated like a broken record stuck on a loop. Whilst I understood the confusion, it was very hard for me to keep explaining things to experts who didn't want to listen.

The ophthalmologist told me to stay on steroid drops long term and when I expressed concern (owing to an increased risk of glaucoma and/or cataracts), I was told that, if I developed cataracts, they would 'whip them out', and this was my only option unless the gastro bods were able to sort out my Crohn's and fistula.

It was pointless trying to explain things and I just nodded and left, unhappy at the prospect of putting steroids into my eyes for the rest of my life. One of the things I used to have on my gratitude list was that I had the gift of sight and now even this was threatened. I really began to believe this nightmare would be the end of me. I just couldn't deal with any more problems. I turned to Dr Google for an explanation of this new problem and it made dire reading and yet again I felt the doctors were missing something. This just didn't add up, but who was I to have an opinion? This whole saga was making me realise just how inconsequential I was.

2018 continued and we were all looking forward to the birth of Annie's second baby, due in September. Cari's birth two years earlier hadn't been straightforward and we were all praying this one would go more smoothly. Cari, my first grandchild, had been born early on in my surgical nightmare and I hadn't been well since she came into the world. This had been a massive disappointment to me as I recall being diagnosed with Crohn's disease when my own daughter was just two years old. It was brutal and made life very difficult. My primal need to look after and protect her gave me the impetus to keep on going at all costs but I would never have managed without my and Andrew's parents. I had hoped that, by the time I had my own grandchildren, if I were lucky enough to survive, my health would be more stable. The heart-breaking thing is that it was, at least until that fateful hysterectomy, when the sleeping dragon within me was awoken and my health was ruined all over again.

Celyn came into the world in September 2018 - she was perfect, and another piece of my heart was totally filled with love and joy. Another difficult birth for Annie which was heart wrenching to witness but all was well in the end, and I felt a deep sense of gratitude and relief. Having been through such a life-changing trauma myself, I viewed everything in life with fear and trepidation, constantly seeking out risks in order to try and mitigate them, which in turn had made me a very anxious and joyless soul.

Things were not to be straightforward, however, when Celyn developed meningitis at just eight weeks old. We were all desperately worried and watching her having cannulas inserted into her tiny hands was just completely heart-breaking. Thankfully she recovered, probably a lot quicker than we did, as it was yet another traumatic experience to witness.

The ongoing therapy was helping Andrew and me but, as my own health continued to be a rollercoaster with more downs than ups, it was a slow process. The fistula felt like a constant threat to my life as it never got significantly better. It sometimes stabilised but then suddenly and without reason, would get much worse, making any sort of normal life impossible. As much as I tried to manage all the problems it brought to my life, I was feeling increasingly lonely and isolated by this awful ailment – a condition that most people had never even heard of.

My consultant had arranged for me to see another colleague who was more local than the London expert. I waited over a year for this to come to fruition, but it was now fast approaching and we were both looking forward to it, yet nervous at the same time. After the attempted repair surgery of 2017, when Andrew watched me almost die from respiratory failure, he was completely opposed to me having more surgery, even though he struggled with life as it was. Like me, he was hoping this new expert could give us some reasons as to why the surgery had gone so wrong and possibly suggest some medication to stabilise things. The eye condition was as debilitating as the fistula in many ways, but I also worried as to what damage the fistula was doing inside. I'd read how they burrow and sometimes I imagined it burrowing through my pelvis like some demonic rodent.

I had met this consultant many times before during my protracted in-patient stay. She was highly thought of and an expert in her field, I really liked her. She was also quite straight-talking without any hint of 'sugar coating' but I had reached a point where I needed some clarity about my options (or lack of them) and I was certainly about to get that.

After taking quite extensive notes, she empathised with me having been cursed with two inflammatory conditions, namely Crohn's disease and endometriosis, as these two together would have caused a lot of damage inside. She also told me that she would not have even attempted to repair the fistula that the original hysterectomy caused, as the risks of making things worse were high, as my repair surgery had shown. She said she generally only attempted repair on people who were already on parenteral nutrition (ie were unable to eat or drink normally and were artificially fed) and as I wasn't in that position, she felt that would have been a big factor in her decision as to whether to operate or not. She also said part of my bladder had been excised in the repair surgery (which possibly explained my constant bladder pain) and the apex of the bladder was now stuck to the fistula. This meant that the removal of the fistula might mean my bladder could be damaged further. There were also no guarantees that further surgery would even work, as the extensive adhesions and inflammation could actually result in more fistulae forming.

It all sounded very disheartening, and I could feel the tears welling up in my eyes. I squeezed Andrew's hand tightly as the disappointment he was feeling was etched in his face and I could tell he too was close to tears. She must have picked up on this and said she wasn't saying it was impossible, but it would be a decision she would not take lightly and I would have to be counselled on the possibility of yet another adverse outcome. She said, if she were to operate, it would mean forming a jejunostomy which basically meant creating an opening at the upper part of the small bowel (the jejunum), providing nutrition artificially at

101

this point whilst the lower part of the small bowel where the fistula was, was removed. The gut would not be re-joined until a few months of healing had passed when a further surgery would be required with the formation of a new stoma further down the digestive tract.

It all sounded pretty terrifying and fraught with danger, and I couldn't imagine ever agreeing to have such extensive surgery again which, apart from anything else, would require months in hospital, miles away from home and my loved ones. My choices were live a half-life with constant problems, enduring a condition that could slowly be killing me, or risk massive surgery which could leave me in a worse position than I was already in, or possibly even death – as this was a possible outcome. More unwelcome news was to follow as she went on to tell me I had gallstones stuck in my common bile duct. I knew this and had been told I needed to get them removed but I had been either too afraid or too unwell. She told me I could not put this off any longer as it could develop into biliary sepsis – a potentially life-threatening condition and more dangerous than the fistula. She said that she would write to my consultant immediately and get this sorted as she would not even consider the fistula until the gallbladder issue was dealt with.

We left in a state of shock, we hadn't been expecting that. We drove home amidst another stony silence yet trying to hold hands at every safe opportunity. What an odd couple we were! I often felt if we could meet in a life without illness, how happy we would be. I just couldn't bear the thought of having to share this news with my family. My mental health was constantly on the edge and I could feel myself retracting into my shell, thereby avoiding the inevitable undesirable and traumatic thoughts which would shortly engulf me yet again. I was unable to discuss or find anything positive in what had been said, only hearing the negatives as usual, not realising that there were many positives on the table too. The prospect of having to go back into that hospital for this gallbladder procedure, which again was not without risk, was just too much to bear and I really did consider if life would be better on the other side.

I hadn't felt so low since this nightmare began. There seemed to be little hope of a repair any time soon and now I had to face going back into hospital to have these errant gallstones removed. The procedure was known as an ERCP - endoscopic retrograde cholangiopancreatography, a procedure that uses endoscopy and X-rays to examine diseases and blockages in the bile ducts - and was not conducted lightly as it was risky. I was absolutely dreading it and my anxiety was off the scale as the trauma of previous surgeries took control of my head.

I was seeing the therapist weekly at this point as she knew I was struggling. She explained how when we experience trauma, our brains don't function like they normally do. We shift into survival mode. Like a deer in the headlights, our brains direct all our mental and physical energy toward dealing with the threat but in my case, there were multiple threats and my brain was constantly seeking them out, trying to mitigate them before they caused more damage to me and my loved ones.

The latest consultation had been too much to process which is why I was feeling so overwhelmed, as if my brain just wanted to disassociate itself from life. As I was trapped in a state of hyper-vigilance, unable to function and think rationally, the therapist suggested I just refused to have the procedure as the anxiety it was causing to me could be more damaging than the small chance of the stones completely blocking the duct. She said she'd write a letter to the consultant.

I was more confused than ever and left the session feeling totally conflicted. I went home and fell asleep, just exhausted by it all. When I awoke, I decided to start the anti-depressants the GP had prescribed months ago. I hadn't taken them when prescribed as I was worried about the side effects. Plus, it was a well-known fact that when you start taking anti-depressant medication, you quite often get worse before improving and I just couldn't risk that.

However, my mental health was deteriorating fast, I just wasn't coping at all and felt fearful at the very black thoughts I was having.

Later than evening, I spoke to a dear friend and she sent me a poem, the saddest thing I've ever read – it was called *The day after I died*. It was a heart-breaking read and reduced me to a blubbering wreck. I promised her I would never ever do such a thing, there was no coming back from that and I would somehow overcome this. Maybe the tablets would help lift my mood. I started them right away and after a few weeks, I did feel brighter and more able to cope. I had obviously become seriously depressed but now a light had gone on, albeit a dim one.

As it happens, when the time came to have the gallbladder procedure, there were no beds and so it was cancelled on the day. All that for nothing! But at least I had started on the medication and did feel slightly more in control and was seeing all the positives in my life, of which there were so many.

Chapter 16

After all the upset and anxiety that the last few months of 2019 had brought, Christmas went surprisingly well and we all had an enjoyable time. My gallbladder and fistula behaved, thank goodness. Since 2015 when my surgery went so badly wrong, Christmas, in keeping with most social events, had become something of a chore, something I was glad to see come and then go. Everything seemed to exhaust me, yet I never felt I could say 'no' for fear of letting people down. Andrew was a gregarious person and enjoyed nothing more than having a houseful of people enjoying themselves. I wanted to do my best for everyone, yet inside I struggled with it all, longing for a quieter life where I was the guest and not the host. It was becoming increasingly apparent that in my quest to protect and support those that I loved so dearly, I had completely and utterly lost myself. But as my friends told me so many times, no one will respect your boundaries if you don't set any. But I never had and had never really wanted to. It was hard to change now but I had little choice.

Early in February 2020, I had a phone call from my mother's care home saying she had a virus and was quite unwell. Fearful of catching anything, I didn't go and see her immediately, something I was to live to regret, but I phoned daily for updates. My sister and daughter visited and commented on her notable weight loss and frailty. She had been this poorly before and we all hoped she would soon pick up again. My sister and daughter had to continue with their everyday lives juggling busy careers, children and running their respective homes, the typical sandwich generation with caring responsibilities at both ends of the age scale. We were lucky insomuch that we were and remain a close family and shared the responsibilities of caring for the old and infirm, as well as the very young members of our family.

A week later, they phoned to say she had been admitted to hospital. The virus had gone to her chest, and she was struggling to breathe. Although I was still worried about catching something, the fact that she'd been admitted to hospital suggested a deterioration in her condition so I knew I had to go to see her. I arrived at the hospital, having bought her the obligatory new nighties and dressing gown, but was shocked at what greeted me. My mother, a previously tall, strong-looking woman, was like a foetal-shaped skeleton in the bed, her chest visibly heaving under the grubby hospital gown. Her eyes had sunk deeply into her head and her hair, now a snowy white, stuck to her forehead as she lay in a pool of sweat, her lips parched and flaky. She was on a busy geriatric ward and they had obviously been trying to feed her which was becoming increasingly difficult. It looked as if she had vomited on her gown and was lying in the mess, making her look grubby and unkempt. No one seemed to have any time for her, with everyone busy on other duties or at break.

I felt sick seeing her and immediately asked to see someone. After a short while, a nurse attended. She explained my mother was very poorly, with a chest infection and pneumonia. She was also dehydrated and her kidneys were failing. This didn't bode well at all. I sat with her and held her tiny hand, her purple veins showing through her thin, translucent skin. She looked up at me and I could see my mother again, her eyes somehow spoke volumes. I felt she knew who I was, and I tried to reassure her that she was safe and loved.

As I spoke those words to her, my heart broke a little more as I thought of how awful her life had been since going into the home, how she did not deserve this, how she was in some ways another casualty of that fateful op of mine. But a voice in my head told me I was wrong and reminded me how we had all tried desperately hard to keep her in her own home and how it had all become just impossible to manage the often-unmanageable world of vascular dementia. After the fire, the care company wouldn't take responsibility for her, so we really had no choice, especially as my own health was on a downward trajectory. I stayed at her bedside for several hours and bathed her parched lips with some wet cotton wool. I fed her ice cream and jelly which she seemed to enjoy. The staff suddenly started to take a bit more notice of her as we put a nice new nightie on her, brushed her hair - she suddenly mattered! My heart broke for all those people who had no one at their side, who could be side-lined because no one cared enough to visit. As I left, the nurse told me the consultant would see me the next day at 2pm when they would explain things in more detail.

We were there promptly at 2 the following day. The consultant was very nice but blunt, my mother's life was coming to an end. By repeatedly pumping her full of antibiotics, we were prolonging the inevitable and her quality of life was diminishing. I told the consultant that I still felt she should be treated, as she had bounced back before. While he respected this, he told me to prepare for the worst, there was only so much her body could take and she had been through so much. We got into a discussion about the futility of prolonging the lives of advanced dementia patients, but I reminded him that primarily, she was our mother and not just another dementia patient. Almost dying alone in a hospital ward myself, where I felt no one believed how I was feeling, was bad enough, but my mother had no means of communicating so we would continue to speak for her. When I got home, I emailed everyone I could think of to see if everything that could be done was being done for her. I asked if she could go into a hospice or a more specialised nursing home, but my pleas were falling on deaf ears although I wouldn't give up on her, ever.

The pneumonia virus that was doing the rounds was brutal and elderly people were, it seemed, particularly vulnerable. My father had died suddenly of pneumonia, aged sixty-four, and I remember then it being referred to as 'the old person's friend', as it carried the sick and infirm to a relatively painless death. My father wasn't old though and I struggled with his cause of death. People in their sixties didn't just die of pneumonia, surely?

But my mother surprised everyone and left hospital a few weeks later, returning to the care home where lots of TLC was prescribed. My sister, daughter and I hatched a plan to visit every day and I looked forward to this time together. She wasn't in pain and was often quite lucid so I hoped our visits would give her some comfort.

An idealised view of how her final weeks would be brought me comfort but more importantly, I prayed that she would somehow know how loved she was and that we hadn't abandoned her. I wanted to get a CD player and play her favourite music, like *I Dreamed a Dream* by Susan Boyle, how she loved that, and *Distant Drums* by Jim Reeves, which would remind her of Dad. I could feed her yogurt and jelly and be the daughter I wanted to be, after years of not fully being there, thanks to the dreaded fistula.

Life, however, had other ideas.

A few days after she came home from hospital, there was a lot of talk on the news about a virus called Coronavirus. It was sweeping the nation and extremely contagious, making people very unwell, even killing them. I couldn't quite believe what I was hearing so chose to blot it out, thinking we were surely safe here in rural West Wales?

Then, without warning, my world was shattered when a call came from the care home, telling me they were closing to visitors until the virus calmed down. I broke down on the phone and said this cannot be happening, she was in the last months of her life but I was told there could be no exceptions. My heart sank as I realised I may never see my mother again.

Within a few days, the Prime Minister had shut the country down for an initial three weeks, much to everyone's shock and horror. I couldn't quite believe what was happening and hoped that at the end of the three weeks, my mother would still be alive and I could see her again and life would get back to normal. But every time I watched the news, my heart sank and those feelings of isolation, fear and massive uncertainty about the future, that had swamped me when my surgery went wrong, came flooding back with a vengeance.

At the start, we embraced it – a daily short walk enabled us to wave at our little granddaughters over their garden wall, often singing songs to them, much to their delight and our embarrassment. My nephews would run up from their house and wait in the garden whilst I made them Nutella pancakes, not allowing them in the house, of course. It was a bit of a game at first but the novelty soon wore off.

As the crisis worsened, my heart broke as I couldn't see the special people in my life, the people who had been my 'armbands' throughout my own trauma. The parks were empty and devoid of the sounds of children's laughter and chatter, the streets I'd walked all my life now empty of friends and acquaintances with whom I'd previously have shared pleasantries or idle chatter. Annie would walk past the house with the children and we would come out to meet, from a safe distance, of course. She would have to hold the girls back so they wouldn't run to us – utter heartbreak. Their little faces showed how much they were failing to understand why they couldn't run to Nanna and Bumpy, as if we were now somehow a danger to them. I'd go back in the house after the precious brief encounter and weep at this unimaginable situation we were in.

And on and on it went..........

There were of course happier moments such as when we held Andrew's sixty-fifth birthday party in the front garden of our bungalow. The rules stated we could not have people indoors but outdoors was fine as long as we kept to the two-metre distance. I got my creative head on and ordered a two-metre caterpillar from Amazon which was made of latex circles. We laid them out on the drive putting a table at either end. We explained to the children they had the head end and we had the bottom end, which they found quite hilarious! I prepared two separate buffets on each table so there was no sharing of anything and the party commenced! The caterpillar was named Fat Bob by Cari and the rules were we had to stick to our respective ends. It turned out to be great fun and everyone enjoyed it. I spoke to many of our neighbours that day, albeit from a distance as they walked past our bungalow for their daily exercise. Neighbours I had never really spoken to before became and remain friends, as did Fat Bob whom we used on many an occasion thereafter.

For me, not having a social life was already normal. My surgical disaster had stopped most of that and foreign holidays were a thing of the past so none of that really affected me. But the pandemic opened up so many wounds for me about how unpredictable life was and brought back the absolute fear of what the future held. I started watching too many news reports and began sinking back into depression.

Ironically, however, seeing and hearing it was OK to recognise the negative emotions people were feeling as the enormity of the pandemic sunk in somehow validated my own negative feelings when my own life had fallen apart. When my surgery had gone wrong, I was plunged into a world of toxic positivity where my negative emotions were discouraged by doctors and even some family members. When I displayed anxiety and depression, I was repeatedly told to be strong, be positive, wise up, stop being self-pitying. But when the pandemic struck and people were experiencing similar emotions of stress, anxiety, and fear at the uncertainty we all faced, we were told these were normal in times of trauma and given coping mechanisms on how to deal with it all! This validated the feelings I had been having about my life-changing experience and allowed me to express and process them. I was no longer alone and I no longer felt my reaction to my trauma was misplaced.

But the monster in my head wasn't going to give up so easily! My coping strategy had been to tell myself if it did happen again, medical help would be available. But then to hear, day after day, stories about people being denied ventilators was just too much. Respiratory failure is pretty terrifying. Please don't try this at home but just imagine taking in a big breath, holding it, then wrapping your head very tightly in cling film so there are no gaps and breathing becomes impossible. The terror in your brain engulfs you as you know death is round the corner unless you get help swiftly. If there is no help, then within a few minutes, you will have a massive heart attack and die.

The thought of there being no help haunted me. I never thought that was even possible in this day and age. I was speaking from the heart of someone in the grips of PTSD. Respiratory failure is so horrific and of course, the very nature of PTSD meant the experience was repeatedly relived through intrusive memories and flashbacks.

I was quite irrational at this point and convinced that if I got the virus and was admitted to hospital with breathing difficulties, I would be denied a ventilator because, after all, once you have an abdominal fistula, you are on borrowed time anyway. I felt sure that if I got Covid and needed a ventilator, I'd be denied one because of my co-morbidities. That's what I believed and no one had told me any different. I decided that if it came to that, I'd sneak in a packet of pills to give myself a swifter ending than suffocating to death. I was so panicked I quite possibly would have taken the pills!

The therapist advised me to stop watching the news so I tried to concentrate on the positives that the pandemic brought. Our little community really came together and I felt a greater sense of connection than previously. Facebook pages were set up by local volunteers where you could talk to someone if you felt down or needed some shopping or medication picking up. It was really heartening to see the community pulling together to support the vulnerable and self-isolating. I continued to do my weekly food shop online. Owing to my underlying health problems, I was very nervous about going out, even for daily exercise but I pushed myself, often resulting in impromptu chats with people I had barely known before. People now made more of an effort to stop and chat and neighbours I barely knew become friends.

I was phoning for regular updates about my mother and was always told she was stable. They seemed more interested in telling me about the lack of PPE or how much pressure they were all under. All true, of course, but I wanted to know how my mother was, was she eating, did she smile or speak, was she free of pain? They said I could come and look at her through an outside window so that's what I decided to do.

A few days later, Andrew drove the short distance to the home and dropped me off. I walked round the back of the building to her room and peeped in the window. Again, all I saw was that foetal-shaped skeletal figure in the bed, her legs contorted. She was alone and her face was emotionless – I tapped the window but she never reacted and this 'meeting' didn't reassure me in any way. I never went back and just prayed the rules could be relaxed as this just seemed inhumane. I blew a kiss through the grubby window pane but somehow, I just knew I'd never see her alive again.

On August 12, 2020, our mother died. The care home for some reason rang my landline. The problem with that was I wasn't home! Andrew had driven me to yet another eye appointment at the hospital ten miles away and left me there whilst he went to pick up something. Luckily, my sister was just a few minutes away from the care home and phoned me. I could tell by her voice it was bad news but of course, I had no means of transport to get back. By the time Andrew arrived back at the hospital and drove me to the home, she had passed. But at least my sister had managed to get there in time to be with her when she passed.

When my mother had left hospital five months ago, we knew she was in her last months of life. One of my concerns was that when her time came, she would not suffer in any way and I was assured she would be given end of life care at the home. This included access to powerful drugs which would be securely stored in a 'just in case' box. These drugs, mainly opioids, would be administered at the end of life when a person started showing signs of distress. But when Covid hit, care homes were no longer permitted to store these drugs and they were returned to the pharmacy. It appears there were no provisions in place should a person deteriorate over the space of a few hours. The care home phoned the surgery several times that morning when my mother started to show signs of distress, but no one was available to come out to her. They sent a prescription to the chemist for the required drugs which arrived two hours after she died. I'm just so glad my sister was there with her but the experience of watching our mother having to gasp for every breath with no help available, left her deeply upset for a very long time thereafter.

Covid got blamed for everything, of course, but to me, it seemed compassion was yet another casualty of the pandemic. My mother hadn't mattered enough, just another old person who died in a home. She didn't get the care she deserved at the end. I just hoped she was blissfully unaware of it all. She was now finally at peace and her suffering over. My feelings were a mixture of guilty relief and absolute gut-wrenching sadness.

The Covid rollercoaster continued. For a while, things improved and we all hoped the end was in sight, only for it all to come crashing down again as things worsened and we were locked down once more. My sixtieth birthday was spent without my close family as my son-in-law-to-be went down with the virus, despite being so cautious. We were all so worried in case Annie got it too as we didn't know what would happen to the children, now aged just four and two. We phoned the helpline and thankfully they told us that, if that happened, a non-vulnerable member of the family would be able to move in to look after the children and my sister volunteered. Yet more 'anticipatory anxiety' that I was now expert at. Yet another parallel with how I felt when I discovered I had a fistula, unable to understand how you can possibly live with a hole in your gut and anticipating death at every twist and turn. Just like now with the entire world facing the prospect of an awfully long fight with an invisible and seemingly invincible enemy, with so many having already lost the fight.

My son-in-law-to-be was fine, Annie and the children didn't get the virus, another period of extreme anxiety over with. I knew I needed to be very careful what I let into my head, as the reality was often very different from what my thoughts told me.

Chapter 17

One year later 2021

The pandemic continued to create so many problems and restrictions, but we plodded on, sticking to the rules, and living within the restrictions.

The fistula continued to be an absolute burden and I never really knew from one week to the next how I would be. If it wasn't a sudden outpouring of blood into the bags or an infection of some kind, it was the inflammatory eye problem which totally wiped me out and sent me to bed. I did, however, have a wonderful new ally in my life, my husband! We had contacted the Royal Naval Association who were very supportive and arranged some one-to-one counselling for him.

After several sessions, he finally let down the shutters and allowed himself to feel all the difficult emotions he'd suppressed for far too long. He was able to express how he regretted encouraging me to have the surgeries, not for one moment expecting this shocking outcome. How he hated his previously strong, funny wife being reduced to a quivering wreck by the constant disappointments life with a fistula dished out. How he was completely worn down by the constant search for support and answers, realising that actually there were no answers, and only my consultant for support. As brilliant as he was, this problem was for life and who could we turn to if he left or retired? But what he regretted most was not believing me and not being there for me 24/7 when I needed him most. Accepting all of this was really hard for both of us but we finally forged a connection that became stronger than ever and that gave me much needed strength and confidence to keep fighting. I finally felt after six long years that he had my back.

As time went on with no real improvement in my condition, the fistula bags themselves now became a problem as I became allergic to them. This was very bad news as a fistula is only as manageable as the bags allow and all of a sudden, mine were not sticking and were causing all sorts of problems. The lovely stoma nurses tried everything, and I spoke to one of my few fistula friends who also had some tricks up her sleeve which she kindly shared with me.

But essentially, the outcome was the same; the bag would only last about six hours before a complete change was required. And of course, the same gut enzymes that would digest a juicy steak were now doing a good job of my skin, making it extremely sore and excoriated, resulting in one awful vicious circle - the worse my skin, the less reliable the bags.

This was really difficult to manage and pushed me into considering whether I should try and have another operation to repair my gut as I just couldn't live like this anymore. Once again, I had become essentially housebound and extremely depressed, despite taking anti-depressants. I was still seeing various doctors but no one really had any solutions. My new gastroenterologist was helpful and was genuinely trying to find answers or at least find something that would improve my quality of life. He suggested I have a sigmoidoscopy whereby a thin tube would be inserted into the rectum to enable them to take some biopsies. If they were able to identify the source of the inflammation, then maybe, just maybe, they would be able to prescribe some medication that could help. That gave me some hope, although with that hope came the fear and trepidation that any hospital procedure now held for me. I'd already had this procedure many times but not since the hysterectomy disaster. On the basis the fistula was situated at the top of the rectum, there were risks attached to the procedure, such as perforation - even the word sent me into a tail spin of anxiety. I said I'd think about it but when I talked to the main surgeon, he said it was too risky. It seemed everything about me was now 'too risky' and how I wished the 'risk-benefit' assessment had had a different outcome when they decided to proceed with the hysterectomy! After living with this for almost seven years, I had come to realise that whilst I am eating, drinking and breathing, I am better off just living with it rather than getting it repaired, as it could so easily make things much worse. My life was to be compromised and difficult but at least I had a life.

Amidst all of this, Annie and her partner had made a very important announcement. They were getting married and the date was set for Easter 2022! I therefore had a very important job to do - helping Annie choose her wedding dress. The first time we went, it was almost a family affair with my sister, Annie's mother-in-law-to-be and the children joining us. Everyone had different thoughts and opinions which added to the mayhem. She decided next time, it would just be the two of us. I told her that when she tried on 'the one' she would know, although she also knew I would provide honest feedback. My face would say it all! We visited several shops, and it was only after several months of searching she finally found one that ticked all the boxes. It was slightly unusual in so much as it had a blush underskirt, and it was beautiful. She almost glided across the floor, and as the sequins and diamantés sparkled in the lights of the bridal boutique, my heart surged with pride and happiness. I couldn't believe the day was finally going to happen, after all the bleakness of the last few years. I felt blessed to be here with Annie and I was so grateful to be sharing the joy of this very special find. I took loads of photos of the dress and the beautiful train which certainly gave it the wow factor. We went for coffee to study the photos in more detail, but she was happy, she had finally said yes to the dress!

All of this was deeply overshadowed by my health, of course, and in particular the leaking bags but I was so grateful and relieved that I'd managed to fulfil my mother of the bride role so far and prayed this would continue to be the case.

My day-to-day life settled into a rather mundane but manageable routine, spent mainly around the house and the children. We would see the girls most days and once a week, we would be on childcare duties with Andrew doing the school runs. The twins would come every day for tea, and we would help with homework if required. Luckily, Andrew is a fount of all knowledge and could be relied upon to provide answers to the most obscure of questions. I was more practical and generally able to help with maths and science when my health and concentration allowed. Last week, whilst trying to grasp the realities of digitised homework with the twins, I actually laughed out loud for the first time in a very long time. Twin One was asking me if there was a God and what did I think of the Big Bang theory? Twin Two was stressing as his laptop wouldn't connect and he had lost all his work, or so he thought. All the while, I was trying and failing to get my head around some algebra question, having never even thought of algebra in about forty-five years! I was becoming increasingly aware of those familiar feelings of 'overwhelm' as they started to flood my brain.

But something changed! I looked at all of us together and instead of collapsing in a heap of despair, I laughed, the twins laughed, we did the algebra, the laptop behaved and Andrew explained the Big Bang theory in way too much detail, resulting in us all putting our heads on the table pretending to snore very loudly.

We finally moved onto Greek mythology homework, and Pandora's Box. This reminded me of an analogy my old gynaecologist had used all those years ago – how by having invasive surgery, I could unleash a prolific source of unwanted troubles, just like the opening of Pandora's Box did. The twins and I talked about how the curious Pandora opened the box, despite being told not to by the gods, and in doing so, unleashed all the evils into the world. When Pandora shut the lid, horrified at what she had done, a small voice called out from within the box, asking to be set free. As Pandora opened the box for a second time, the little bug was freed. 'I am Hope,' it said, 'and whilst I am in the world, you will be able to muster up the courage to live through bad times and hope for better days.'

The twins looked at me and asked, 'What does that mean, Aunty?' I explained that, in the midst of all the troubles in the world, there is always hope and that is what will ultimately get us through.

Chapter 18

2022

As 2021 drew to a close, I realised the wedding would soon be upon us and I was reminded daily by the countdown timer carefully placed on the freezer door in my kitchen. A few days after New Year, private messages started coming through about hen party options – from boozy weekend breaks to afternoon teas, all completely out of my comfort zone. My first thought was there was just no way I could attend any of these events; Annie would understand if I wasn't there.

I had, however, realised some time ago, that sometimes it's very easy to become trapped by those feelings. It somehow felt safer to be unhappy as then there was no risk of disappointment, a sort of very unhealthy comfort blanket. In the early days of the fistula, any sign of healing sent me into a feeling of almost euphoria as I convinced myself the nightmare was ending. I'd be ordering handbags and booking holidays, only for my world to come crashing down a few weeks later when it inevitably burst open with the spectacular goriness that only a fellow sufferer or medic would understand. I found it easier not to be hopeful or happy as the seemingly inevitable disappointments that life with a fistula brings were just too painful. I'd rather remain in the much safer place called Gloomsville, thank you very much. But misery begets misery and I found my low mood risked permeating into the souls of everyone that mattered to me. Now was my chance to break free of this prison and try and find a new perspective where I could be happy despite the fistula. I couldn't carry this sadness around forever, the burden was too heavy and it had already broken me more than once.

So I was one of the first to accept the hen party invitation, much to my sister's surprise. As Chief Bridesmaid, she was arranging it and her choice of party took my problems into account. I bought a new outfit and started on a strict diet to try and lose the 25lbs I had gained in recent years. Remember misery begets misery, I had become so sad, stopped caring, stopped looking in the mirror at my horrific body and as a consequence, to add to my problems, I developed a weight problem. But this was my chance to sort my act out and get back to living my life, maybe not the one I'd hoped for, but a precious, beautiful life nonetheless, occasionally sprinkled with fun!

But once again, the fistula had other plans and seemed determined to drag me back down to the bottomless pit. A few days into January, I started losing blood. I was sitting on the bed while Andrew was in the front room, watching a film in a kind of post-Christmas slump. I'd been to the toilet and noticed blood in my fistula bag. Nothing unusual in the appearance but the quantity was more than I was comfortable with. I sat on the bed and prayed it would settle, only to feel a warm sensation under my bottom. I soon realised I was bleeding from there too, and from my stoma, and from the fistula hole that had previously closed! I looked down to see my abdominal wall pouring with blood like beetroot juice through a colander. I called Andrew and had a grumpy 'WHAT NOW?' in reply. He hated me calling him as he knew it meant one of two things. Either I was ill, or I needed a job doing, both of which he no longer relished dealing with.

He came into the bedroom and looked visibly shocked. The blood was now dripping down the edge of the bed onto the grey fluffy rug. Fortunately, my son-in-law-to-be arrived at that point and thankfully took control, telling Andrew to call an ambulance. He asked me if I had eaten lots of beetroot which made me smile, secretly hoping that I would suddenly remember the two jars I'd eaten lunch time but of course, that wasn't the case. I'd never eat beetroot for that very reason. Andrew came back in the room and said the ambulance would be six hours and he had to drive me himself. I don't think I'd felt so vulnerable since that awful night seven years ago when my bowel had perforated and there were no beds at the hospital. I was gripped with fear then and those feelings returned with a vengeance. Andrew got me in the car and I sat on a pile of towels, me as ever the practical one, worrying about damaging the car's upholstery.

We're not the type to make a fuss but on this occasion, he went into A&E and said I was in the car bleeding, and he needed help. When they saw me, I think they thought I'd been shot as I was gripping my stomach to try and keep the blood in the bags, without much success. I managed to walk in accompanied by a nurse, followed by a trail of blood. I was swiftly taken to a bay and hooked up to several drips including saline and a clotting drug. Andrew was not allowed to stay with me and waited in the car for news. A CT was arranged, and a bed was found. The blood still poured from every available orifice, black sticky blood that stained my fingers and got in deep under my nails. It gave off a sickly-sweet metallic smell that made me gag, but as the clotting drug took hold, it began to resemble red cottage cheese.

I was, however, very well looked after and saw many doctors, all of whom looked quite shocked at the state of my abdomen. Three bags had now been filled, albeit more slowly, with dark red blood, yet the CT provided no real answers. There was no evidence of any active bleed. My observations were reasonably ok, although I had developed a high temperature and my haemoglobin level had dropped from a routine blood test I'd coincidentally had a few days before. I drifted in and out of sleep, quite secure in the knowledge they were keeping a close eye on things.

I stayed in hospital for five days and was discharged without any real explanation of what had happened. I had been taking ibuprofen for my eye condition and they felt that could have been a contributory factor, but they weren't sure. I'd had a pelvic MRI to check there was no active bleed anywhere else and I was told they'd write to me with the results.

I arrived home feeling like I'd been hit by a train and didn't even have the energy to have a shower. I slept for about eighteen hours and woke up in an awful mess. On days like this, I knew I needed more help but with the whole world catching up following Covid, there was just nowhere to go for that help.

A few days later, I felt better and tried not to dwell on that event, terrifying as it was. With renewed energy, I stepped on the scales - and had lost six pounds! Every cloud and all that . . .

The weeks passed and the hen party was getting nearer. The outfit I'd bought fitted better, due to my weight loss. It was a dark colour with strategically-placed pockets to enable me to have a reassuring 'tap tap tap' on my abdomen to ensure all was ok and nothing was leaking. Although I was becoming increasingly nervous at the prospect of going out, I knew I had to go through with it or I would be a prisoner to this demon forever. Andrew had agreed to pick me up after the meal so I would only actually be out of the house for five hours. The rest of the group were going to a cocktail bar and then on to watch the Wales v England rugby match. The fact Andrew had agreed to miss the first half of such a big game to pick me up was quite a rarity, as I've always come second to rugby, but he too felt secretly nervous at the prospect of me going 'out out', especially without him.

The Party Bus arrived on the town square, belting out Abba tunes at full blast. I realised it must have been my sister's choice of music as she loves Abba. As I smiled at this thought, I spotted her walking from the rugby club with a bottle of Asti in hand, closely followed by the rest of the group including the bride-to-be, my daughter, dressed up in a veil, tiara and bride-to-be glasses. I sat in the car and felt frozen with fear, preferring the prospect of a quiet day at home on my own in front of the TV. Again! But no, I decided to take the plunge and walked the few steps to the bus where I was greeted with lots of noise and clapping as they were surprised to see me. I sat next to my sister-in-law and soon we were off! In a short while, we were all singing exuberantly to *Delilah* on the karaoke machine and I actually felt relaxed and happy for the first time in a very, very long time.

It took about an hour to get to the restaurant and I suspected things would go downhill a little now as I would have to eat in public, something I still struggled with. My meal arrived and it was a massive plate of beige coloured pasta which I picked at while trying to talk to everyone else. A few people commented on the fact I wasn't eating much but it went largely unnoticed. It's frustrating as I was actually ravenous but had I eaten more than a few mouthfuls, the fistula would have sprung into action and completely stressed me out. The afternoon passed quickly and I did enjoy a small glass of wine and a coffee. Soon it was 4pm and Andrew arrived to take me home. I said my goodbyes and got in the car feeling so happy at my accomplishment. I looked at Annie as I was leaving and she looked beautiful and radiant and I felt more confident about the wedding that was now just six weeks away.

On Mother's Day, we decided to have an afternoon tea in the garden. We bought most of the food, including a cake to save me cooking. Our guests arrived around 4pm on a lovely sunny afternoon. The children played and the adults chatted and it all went really well. But I wasn't feeling great, exceptionally tired and with a strange irritating cough. I went to bed that night, totally wiped out to the point I couldn't even clean up after our do, leaving that to Andrew to sort out.

I awoke at 3am shivering and I knew I had a fever which the thermometer told me was 39 degrees. In the morning, I did a lateral flow test and yes, I had Covid. So, after two years of being exceptionally cautious and dodging it, I now had the dreaded virus just a couple of weeks before the wedding, with Andrew testing positive a few days later.

I sent a message on our family group chat, telling everyone our news. We would isolate for the required time which meant we would miss our friend's wedding the following weekend, which disappointed us enormously. After a few days, however, I began to relish the opportunity to rest and relax. I didn't have to cook or clean and could spend my days watching TV and doing very little without feeling guilty. Initially Andrew had no symptoms and so painted all the fencing outside as he felt he had to keep busy. He was worried that, as in the first wave, on day 9 or 10, we would suddenly deteriorate and require hospitalisation. I tried to reassure him that things were different now, as we were triple-vaccinated for starters and serious illness was thankfully now quite rare. He wasn't convinced though and after a few days, he did indeed get worse, feeling short of breath and generally unwell. Or maybe he was fed up with fence painting? Whatever the reason, he too dropped anchor and chilled out. We quite enjoyed this welcome break, if truth be known, where life stopped and we took time for each other for once. By about day ten, we were both testing negative and went to town for coffee, which was a welcome treat. With the wedding now just ten days hence, we had a lot of catching up to do. I had a hat to pick up and shoes to buy, yet still I found doing anything just wiped me out, which seems a typical after effect of Covid.

A week before the wedding, Andrew awoke with a swollen tongue, of all things. If Fate couldn't get me, it was obviously going to go for my husband! This really was going to be a tough race to the finish, and I did wonder what else would be chucked at us. He spent several hours at the hospital being pumped full of steroids in case he was having an allergic reaction to something. Again, they weren't really sure what the cause was but his tongue became so swollen at one point, he couldn't speak properly and he worried about being able to deliver his Father of the Bride speech.

The steroid injection seemed to do the trick, luckily, and he was prescribed oral steroids and antihistamines for a few days as a 'just in case'. With a busy week ahead, this was the last thing we needed but we plodded on and as every day passed, my feelings of excitement and anxiety built. Annie was understandably exceptionally busy and I worried about her as I knew she wasn't sleeping well but I soon had to put that to one side, as Fate had yet another go at us and Andrew developed severe toothache! This required an emergency dental appointment and a large dose of antibiotics.

The stress was starting to get to me but I managed to control it and told myself repeatedly it would all be wonderful.

The night before the wedding finally arrived, the tongue had returned to normal, the toothache was being controlled by pain killers and we were trying very hard to relax. I'd had my hair done and my nails polished, my outfit had been taken over to Annie's as I was getting dressed there with the bridesmaids and the bride, of course. We had a grazing breakfast board arriving at 9am and the Bucks Fizz was chilling nicely. I really didn't want to miss out, I wanted it to be like before the fistula, when I felt normal and complete, excited at just being alive.

I took extra care doing my bags that night, carefully warming them on the radiator to make the adhesive stickier. This time last year, I was having a complete nightmare with my bags, and constant leakages had left me almost housebound. I'd met a girl on Facebook who has an abdominal fistula. She told me about the bags she used and showed me how she applied them. I ordered some samples, took her advice and have never looked back. They have helped so much and I remain so grateful to her for taking the trouble to help me out, despite her own health battles, of which there are many.

Andrew helped me apply the bags as usual and we went to bed saying a silent prayer for everything to be ok. This was to be a massive milestone for me and it just had to go well.

We awoke at about 8am to a stream of sunshine that had sneaked in through a gap in the curtains. It looked like a lovely day out there. Andrew brought me a cup of tea as he does every day and I was relieved to see his face hadn't swelled up as he'd feared. He'd asked me to walk Annie down the aisle if he hadn't been able to attend, but for once, it was me telling him, 'You will be fine.' The shoe was on the other foot now and I wasn't used to seeing this fear and vulnerability in him. It somehow made me stronger and more determined that this day would go well. My heart was pounding in my chest as I thought I detected a leak on one of the bags, but a cursory 'tap tap tap' told me all was well, just the fistula demon testing my resilience again. It would, of course, be disastrous to have to change the bags now as they take several hours to settle, time I didn't have this morning. A leaking fistula bag was most certainly not an option.

We drove the two-minute journey to Annie's house where I walked into happy chaos with the photographer and video man standing about waiting to capture the morning. My heart stopped as I glanced in the lounge to see youngest granddaughter Celyn covered in chocolate after eating a gooey muffin, most of which seemed to be on the floor precariously close to where The Dress hung in all its splendour.

The children were ushered out of the lounge and sent upstairs to watch a film for half an hour with the eldest flower girl in charge. Make up was being done, and hair coiffed, and it all seemed to be coming together just perfectly. I still felt terribly anxious and the lovely hair lady made me a coffee to calm me down. I then progressed to Bucks Fizz and nibbles and started to feel more relaxed and actually enjoyed the beautiful chaos as it unfolded before me. I was probably being fuelled by adrenaline as I had butterflies in my stomach constantly. Time was getting on though and I could feel tensions rising as we really should be dressed by now - children first, then the bridesmaids. I, at this point, was still in my dressing gown, too scared to see if the Buck's Fizz and nibbles had caused any reaction but fortunately all was fine. The make-up girl helped me with my dress, she was so kind, her eyes tactfully looking away at the sight of my battered body.

I remember the psychiatrist telling me, a few years back, that I would hopefully eventually reach a point where, rather than see myself as mutilated and broken, I'd see myself as a survivor, as one who manages the often unmanageable. I would come through stronger, more resilient, on the other side. I looked in the mirror and my first thought was, 'I wish I'd said no to the daily chocolate bar.' I was heavier than I wanted to be but so what? This is me, I am what I am, take me or leave me. But I knew this confidence wouldn't last.

Annie looked radiant. The dress and the beautiful train seemed much harder to handle in the confines of her hallway and as she struggled to get her earrings in, I couldn't get close to her to help for fear of standing on it. Finally, she was ready. A last-minute panic erupted when one of the cats escaped but was miraculously caught by one of the bridesmaids and returned to a place of safety. The vintage cars had already arrived and sparkled in the spring sunshine, ready to take us to the church and then onto the reception at Sylen Lakes, a beautiful location nestled at the foot of Mynydd Sylen in Carmarthenshire.

It turned into the most magical, perfect, happy day. The sun shone as brightly as Annie's smile and everything went to plan. I remembered my daughter, as a little girl, would refuse to leave the house if her shoes weren't perfectly clean and laces symmetrical. It was quite a challenge at times but that meticulous personality paid off as the planning of every detail of the wedding had come to fruition perfectly. I disappeared to the lodge at 5 o clock to check my bags and to have a lie down. The lodge was on the side of the lake and was as beautiful as everything else. I sat at the picnic tables and my nephew made me a cup of tea. I took my shoes off and breathed in the fresh air, my skin warmed by the afternoon sun. I felt relaxed and so grateful everything had gone well. I went to check my bags and they were fine, so I decided to leave them. I knew I wouldn't be eating again that day and my dancing and drinking days were done, so hopefully they would last until we got home. We returned to the reception, and I realised life could be good again – today had been testament to that.

Chapter 19

Adapting to life with a disability or chronic illness is an emotional rollercoaster. Despite the fact I'd first experienced ill health in my twenties, this was different in so many ways. The stoma I'd had all those years ago in my twenties was planned and restored my health, whereas the complications caused by the hysterectomy had taken it all away again and robbed us of our future dreams and hopes. Plus, of course, it was an unexpected complication - one that was rare, permanent and life changing - so it was a massive shock which we had to deal with, whilst normal life crumbled around us with the ripple effects spreading wide and far. I somehow expected someone to turn up and say, 'Don't worry, this can be easily fixed.' But no one said that it was always watch, wait and hope. One nurse said to me, 'Well, you signed the consent form, this is a risk of abdominal surgery.' I found that very harsh and thought if someone had got into a car and had a horrific accident, you wouldn't say, 'Well, you made the decision to get in the car.' It all seemed so callous and so terribly isolating, besides which I never in a million years expected this to happen.

The psychological effects of surgical complications are huge, due to delayed recovery or, in my case, a long-lasting disability. It is, of course, well documented how stress delays wound healing and even compromises immunity. You would think, therefore, more help would be available to consider the psychological effect of these life-changing complications with a view to offering support and information to the patient at the most vulnerable time of their life. I found almost the opposite happened – the outcome was often played down and normalised as if it was of no great significance, and I just had to accept it all. I understand most complications are nowhere near as serious as mine and most surgeries happen with no significant problems. It just seems that there are no mechanisms in place when these rare events do happen. Had there been, maybe I would have managed my expectations better - for years, I expected to heal but I was knocked back time and time again which added to my trauma. I learned in time this type of fistula cannot heal spontaneously (unless it does so in the first few months), it had to be surgically removed, which in my case, was probably too dangerous.

The journey to acceptance can mirror the five-stage grieving process as grief isn't limited to the death of a loved one, but also the loss of your health and of the life you once lived and loved. I can certainly identify to all the five stages, starting with denial. I had a complete inability to accept the situation and convinced myself it would heal, as the alternative just was not an option. It was a way of avoiding reality for a while, as it was less traumatic for me, maybe a kind of inbuilt defence mechanism.

Next came anger – I have certainly displayed a lot of anger over the years, directed at myself and my loved ones, especially my husband. I became an extremely angry and unhappy person as the reality of my situation sunk in.

Bargaining is another stage and another way that our brains process what has happened. You believe that it was all an awful mistake and you could somehow turn the clock back, or you try to negotiate with God to make it all go away and the trauma end, in return for becoming a better person.

Then comes depression which completely swamped me, to a point I could not accept life with the fistula. It was just too awful, too unpredictable and too traumatic for me to live with. The depression took away all positives from life to the point where I could find no pleasure in anything. I was so damaged that I lived my life in a state of permanent anxiety, waiting for the next disaster to happen. I had to resort to medication in the end which did lift the blackness somewhat and enabled me to see what I still had and what I could still do despite my situation. The depression still lingers and any flare up of problems reignites the trauma, causing me to nose dive. I must keep a very close eye on myself these days. I am learning to say no, take a step back, pace myself and put myself first and if people don't like it, then they quite simply aren't my people.

Finally, and hopefully, comes acceptance. This is the stage where you can see a life with your particular disability or illness. For the first five or six years, life with the dreaded fistula just wasn't an option, it had to go. But in year seven, I did begin to accept what had happened, because life was just passing me by. I realised I would have to make some changes to make my new life manageable but it was possible, my life was not over.

There are still so many times when I grieve deeply for the life I have lost, mainly because I have to deal with Andrew's disappointment, as he had big plans for our future as regards travel etc. I went through a phase of feeling this was somehow avoidable, it just shouldn't have happened. It wasn't an Act of God or a terrible accident, it was a conscious decision I made (with much trepidation, I add), fuelled by the guidance of my much-trusted surgeons, which had the most terrible, permanent consequences. I blamed myself, the surgeons, my husband, anyone, and everyone - but of course this was all futile. I spent years looking for answers that didn't exist, writing to specialists all over the country who often never even replied - desperate to find something - anything - that could undo the damage and take me back to a life when my body enabled me to live normally again. However, this constant search for answers actually had the reverse effect - and just like a snowball increasing in size as it races down a snowy bank, the trauma grew and became entrenched in my mind, until I could no longer function.

After a long search, I found a professional who specialised in counselling those who have experienced difficult or traumatic experiences in healthcare. She explained the concept of 'Second Harm' whereby there was a poor institutional response to serious surgical outcomes like mine. Second Harm reduced the chances of those who have experienced harm returning to functionality, and prolongs and exacerbates the harm caused by the initial event. Whilst my consultant had been very supportive, there was little support elsewhere, and I was too weak and damaged to challenge or question anyone, let alone professionals. However, after many months of therapy, I started to see the light again and realised there was much more to life that the darkness of the past couldn't take away.

Thanks to Linda, I developed a confidence and strength that had been demolished, until I finally realised I was enough and ready to move on with whatever life had in store for me.

I still live with many debilitating problems - two stoma bags, bladder problems, eye problems and great deal of uncertainty - but my PTSD-fuelled fear of the future has to be beaten into submission every day to enable me to live again and make it the best life I can, despite the fistula. Moving forward, I wish myself (and everyone else managing these invisible, sometimes impossible conditions), a big pot of courage, a tower of strength, a bucket full of love and an abundance of hope – oh, and of course, an unwavering determination to dance in the rain, at least some of the time.

Acknowledgments

Sharp Scratch started as a journal, written from my hospital bed, to consume the time during my protracted hospital stays. Thanks to many people, it is now a book, a book that has connected me with other people in a similar situation, providing mutual comfort, support and inspiration.

I would like to express my deepest gratitude to the following who have helped me in so many different ways -

Firstly, my publisher Penny Reeves of Saron Publishers, without whom this book would not have happened. Penny has been extremely supportive and patient from the outset which, considering my inexperience and limited IT skills, has been extremely welcome and much needed!

Very special thanks to my precious nearest and dearest who have been there for me through all my years of surgeries. It's because of you that I keep going, determined to live life with contentment and joy from here on in, no matter what.

To my friends – old friends, new friends, cyber friends and forever friends - thank you. You have listened, supported and been there for me through everything and I'm eternally grateful to you all. Too many to mention for fear of missing someone out but you know who you are.

To Dr. Linda Kenward, Integrative Counsellor MBACP – I first read about Linda a few years ago. She specialises in helping people who have experienced adverse outcomes in a healthcare setting. She has been a massive support to me, allowing me to process my feelings without judgement, granting me the freedom of acceptance and the ability to move on. I am forever grateful, Linda.

To the many wonderful doctors (and secretaries), nurses and stoma nurses out there who have provided unwavering support throughout.

And last but in no way least, thanks to Barney, my floppy eared goon of a dog, who every evening comes and sits on my feet, keeping them warm and making me smile.

Helpful Resources

Websites and Facebook pages which I've found helpful:

Facebook groups

Abscess/Fistula support for women

Enterocutaneous Fistula Support Group

UK Sepsis Trust Support Group

Ileostomy & Stoma Support group

https://www.facebook.com/FistulaAwareness

Websites

https://crohnsandcolitis.org.uk (Crohns and Colitis organisation)

https://gutscharity.org.uk (Guts uk)

https://iasupport.org (Ileostomy Association)

https://www.menopausematters.co.uk

Author Bio

Deborah Jay was born and raised in West Wales. She married aged twenty and moved to Plymouth with her Chief Petty Officer husband. The Falklands War started shortly after, meaning her husband went on a long commission, resulting in her returning home to her beloved Carmarthenshire where she raised their only child. She worked for twenty-five years in Local Government before retiring owing to her declining health. Her life now revolves around her family, friends and pet dog. She has always had a love of writing and has penned a few children's books for her beloved grandchildren and nephews, which they loved.

Sharp Scratch, however, is her first published book at the grand old age of 62!

Printed in Great Britain
by Amazon